Occupational Therapy Stories: Psychosocial Interaction in Practice

Occupational Therapy Stories: Psychosocial Interaction in Practice

Barbara Borg, MA, OTR
Colorado State University
Fort Collins, Colorado

Mary Ann Bruce, MS, OTR
Independent Contractor
Irvine, California

SLACK Incorporated, 6900 Grove Road, Thorofare, NJ 08086-9447

Publisher: John H. Bond
Editorial Director: Amy E. Drummond
Associate Editor: Jennifer J. Cahill
Creative Director: Linda Baker

Borg, Barbara.

Occupational therapy stories: psychosocial interaction in practice/Barbara Borg, Mary Ann Bruce.

p. cm.

Includes bibliographical references and index.

ISBN 1-55642-313-6

1. Occupational therapy—Case studies. 2. Occupational therapy—Problems, exercises, etc. I. Bruce, Mary Ann. II. Title.

[DNLM: 1. Mental Disorders—therapy—case studies. 2. Occupational Therapy—case studies. 3. Occupational Therapy—problems. WM 450.5.02B732o 1997]

RC487.B67 1997
616.89'14—dc21
DNLM/DLC
for Library of Congress 96-53891

Printed in the United States of America

Published by: SLACK Incorporated
6900 Grove Road
Thorofare, NJ 08086-9447 USA
Telephone: 609-848-1000
Fax: 609-853-5991

Contact SLACK Incorporated for more information about other books in this field or about the availability of our books from distributors outside the United States.

Last digit is print number: 10 9 8 7 6 5 4 3 2 1

Dedication

To Andrew, Juan Carlos, John, and to Emily,
who reminds us to see the eagle within.

Contents

INTRODUCTION

CHAPTER 1: THERAPEUTIC RELATIONSHIP

CHAPTER 2: ESTABLISHING TRUST

CHAPTER 3: ASSESSING SAFETY

Key Topics: Allen's cognitive disability model; cognitive levels; Allen Cognitive Level test; safety and guardianship; Kohlman Evaluation of Living Skills; discharge planning

CHAPTER 4: PROFESSIONAL BOUNDARIES

Key Topics: Ego function; psychodynamically based occupational therapy; dissociative identity disorder; using art in therapy; responding to suicidal behavior; therapist privacy; documentation; reimbursement for service

CHAPTER 5: CONFUSED BEHAVIOR

Key Topics: Kaplan's directive group; psychosis; reality testing; delusional system; safety concerns; helping client group respond to confused behavior

CHAPTER 6: AGGRESSIVE BEHAVIOR

Key Topics: Threatening behavior; adolescence; conduct disorder; safety; therapeutic milieu

CHAPTER 7: QUALITY OF LIFE

Key Topics: The wish to die; manipulation; quality of life; adult development issues; integrity versus despair; chronic pain; pain management; caretaking; educating staff

CHAPTER 8: NORMAL DEVELOPMENT

Key Topics: Client expectations; therapist as expert; traumatic brain injury; emotional changes in acquired brain impairment; holism; developmental issues with the younger client; parent concerns; medical ethics

CHAPTER 9: COMMUNITY CONTEXT

Key Topics: Behavior modification; extinguishing behavior; traumatic brain injury; social skills training; modeling; cognitive strategies; community reentry; family's role and expectations

CHAPTER 10: PERSONAL MEANING OF OBJECTS

Key Topics: Objects and their meaning; depression; grief; lost and misplaced belongings; role of family in treatment; behavior modification; behavioral frame of reference; disengagement; role of occupational therapy with terminally ill clients

CHAPTER 11: REENGAGEMENT

Key Topics: Occupational therapy outreach to homeless persons; community reentry; older adult; responding to withdrawn individual; grief; symbolic communication; the arts in occupational therapy

CHAPTER 12: AWARENESS OF CHANGE

Key Topics: Alzheimer's dementia; anxiety; family denial; cognitive frameworks for occupational therapy practice; functional approach; dynamic interactional model; objects as cognitive organizers and links to identity and purpose; metacognition

CHAPTER 13: DISABILITY AND THE FAMILY

Key Topics: Family dynamics and working with families; treatment planning and goal setting with families; traumatic brain injury; cognitive impairment; personality change; spousal abuse; establishing competence; return to work; return to home; driver training; financial management

CHAPTER 14: CLIENT PERCEPTIONS

Key Topics: Changes in self-perception; personal standards; depression; traumatic brain injury; grounded theory; adjusting to disability; community reintegration; community treatment programs; dependence; family education; individualizing treatment; performance feedback; journaling; spousal support

Acknowledgments

We wish to express our appreciation to the occupational therapists who contributed their stories: Martina M. Cooper, Mary E. Conrad, Susy Stark, and those who preferred to remain anonymous. We have learned immeasurably from the glimpses given into both the therapist and client experience. We are grateful to the artist/friend who enhanced our understanding of the power of the bear, and we thank Kevin and Polly for allowing us to share and comment on their personal story.

Working with the editorial staff at SLACK Incorporated has been a pleasure. We thank John Bond, Amy Drummond, and Jennifer Cahill for their enthusiastic support of this project. We appreciate their trust in us, and the helpful suggestions they made that guided us in the final drafting of this text.

About the Authors

Barbara Borg, MA, OTR, has a bachelor's degree in occupational therapy from Colorado State University and a master's degree in counseling psychology from the University of Northern Colorado. She has engaged in occupational therapy practice and in individual, couple, family, and group counseling, consultation, and education with children and adults of all ages. She has held the position of Director of Occupational Therapy and Field Work Coordinator at Bethesda Hospital in Denver, Colorado, and for many years was part of the Colorado Council on Basic Education. She is currently Assistant Professor at Colorado State University, where she has taught for 8 years, and has also served as affiliate faculty. While teaching, she has maintained a small practice. In 1995, she received the Gilfoyle Award for Teaching Excellence.

Barbara's articles have appeared in the *American Journal of Occupational Therapy*, and she has been a presenter at national and state professional conferences. She has been a reviewer for the *American Journal of Occupational Therapy* and *Occupational Therapy Journal of Research*, and served on the Editorial Board for the American Occupational Therapy Association's *Cognitive Rehabilitation: Self-Study Series* (1993). She and Mary Ann Bruce have co-authored two other books in the area of psychosocial practice: *The Group System: The Therapeutic Activity Group in Occupational Therapy* (1991) and *Psychosocial Occupational Therapy: Frames of Reference for Intervention* (1987, 1993). Barbara and Mary Ann also contributed a chapter to *Occupational Therapy: Overcoming Human Performance Deficits* (Christiansen & Baum, 1991).

Barbara lives in Colorado with her two children, Andrew and Emily.

Mary Ann Bruce, MS, OTR, completed her bachelor's degree in occupational therapy and home economics at Colorado State University and her master's degree in counseling at Southern Connecticut State University. She is currently completing a doctorate in educational psychology at the University of Southern California. She has pursued her interests in mental health, cognition, learning, group and community intervention, and administration in occupational therapy practice, education, consultation, and scholarly activities. Since beginning her career in 1967, some of her positions have included: Director of Occupational Therapy at Bethesda Hospital and Community Mental Health Center, Denver, Colorado; Associate Professor and Chairperson of Occupational Therapy at Quinnipiac College, Hamden, Connecticut; and Associate Professor and Interim Chairperson of Occupational Therapy at the University of Texas Health Science Center, San Antonio. She has assumed professional responsibilities as an accreditation site visitor for the American Occupational Therapy Association, reviewer for the *American Journal of Occupational Therapy*, reviewer of several AOTA Self-Study projects, and test writer for specialty certification exams. Currently, she is an independent contractor in occupational therapy in Irvine, California.

Mary Ann's current teaching and research focus is motivation, learning strategies, cognitive processing, and problem solving.

Overview of Chapters

CHAPTER 1: THERAPEUTIC RELATIONSHIP

Jane is a woman in her 50s dealing with chronic obstructive pulmonary disease, fibromyalgia, and possibly a paranoid disorder. The therapist strives to establish a therapeutic alliance with Jane, who antagonizes many of her caregivers and tells the therapist that she has been mistreated.

CHAPTER 2: ESTABLISHING TRUST

Marilyn is a depressed older woman who has been voluntarily admitted for psychiatric treatment to an inpatient facility. She now fears that she and other patients are getting "worse" and that she cannot leave the treatment setting.

CHAPTER 3: ASSESSING SAFETY

Ben has mild, unspecified dementia. The therapist uses Allen's cognitive disability model to help determine what will be a safe living environment for Ben.

CHAPTER 4: PROFESSIONAL BOUNDARIES

Sally is a young woman with two distinct personalities. She does well in a supportive, psychodynamically oriented program and is discharged. Then a crisis occurs, and the therapist is called at home.

CHAPTER 5: CONFUSED BEHAVIOR

Kathy, a confused middle-aged patient, wanders into the occupational therapy group. The therapist describes her actions and how she feels uncomfortable knowing that she is part of someone's delusional belief system.

CHAPTER 6: AGGRESSIVE BEHAVIOR

Frankie is an angry 17-year-old male with conduct disorder who physically threatens the therapist. The therapist describes her responses and those of a very frightened patient group.

CHAPTER 7: QUALITY OF LIFE

Mr. Callahan is an older adult who has been wealthy and influential in his community. Physical pain and impaired vision have decreased his independence and ability for everyday enjoyment, and he asks the therapist, "(Is it) morally wrong to kill yourself?"

The narrator describes a luncheon meeting with Anita, a woman whose back pain makes it difficult for her to sit for anything but brief periods. This woman asks, "Is life worth living?"

In "Leave Me Alone," a 93-year-old woman, debilitated and recovering from a hip fracture, wants staff to leave her alone and let her die.

CHAPTER 8: NORMAL DEVELOPMENT

Jeff is a high school sophomore whose world has been turned upside down by a skateboard injury. Although Jeff is cooperative, the therapist recognizes that his compliance may counter a healthy adolescent need for independence.

CHAPTER 9: COMMUNITY CONTEXT

Treatment staff are asked to implement a behavior modification program with Nathan following his traumatic brain injury. Carrying this program out in the community creates practical problems and philosophical concerns for the therapist.

CHAPTER 10: PERSONAL MEANING OF OBJECTS

In "The Dress," an older woman discovers that her favorite dress has been lost by staff where she is in transitional care. She grieves this and many other losses.

In "Objects d'Art," a woman lawyer in her 40s no longer seems motivated to participate in therapy following her cerebral vascular accident. The family wants to help her continue, but is uncertain as to what will motivate her.

Having been told she is terminally ill, Leah sells or gives away most of her belongings to enter a nursing facility. Then the story changes.

CHAPTER 11: REENGAGEMENT

A woman with a history of schizophrenia enters a homeless shelter depressed, withdrawn, and mourning the death of her two grown sons. A trip to the city art museum brings some startling results.

CHAPTER 12: AWARENESS OF CHANGE

The therapist is called to simplify Glenn's routine and hopefully decrease his anxiety. During a visit, he struggles to sing the therapist a poignant song from the opera *Pagliacci*.

CHAPTER 13: DISABILITY AND THE FAMILY

Dr. D. has been a successful physician. When he experiences a head trauma, his wife assumes greater responsibility within the family. His return home and imminent return to employment upset family dynamics.

CHAPTER 14: CLIENT PERCEPTIONS

Kevin is a young man whose life is radically changed by head injury. He chronicles his feelings about himself, his beliefs, and his therapy experiences in two journals that span 3 years. His wife, Polly, recounts her wish to understand and support Kevin.

INTRODUCTION

Our First Story

An instructor tells her class: "When my daughter Emily was 4 years old, she was determined that she would someday be an eagle; not just any eagle, but a great eagle. She would tell me, 'I'll fly away, Mommy, but sometimes I'll come back and spread my wings and take you on my back, anywhere you want to go.' It was, for me, a wonderful image, so full of possibility. I'd hear her friends in the neighborhood say that when they grew up they were going to be 'a mommy,' but Emily would always reply matter-of-factly, 'I'm going to be an eagle.' Each time I'd overhear her say this, I was secretly pleased. Then one day, she came home from school and announced, 'You know what happened today? My class talked about what we were going to be when we grew up and I said I was going to be an eagle. But my teacher said I couldn't be an eagle. She said I would have to be a "lady"...And all the kids laughed at me.' Unsure of how to respond, I turned to her and asked 'So, then, what do you think?' Emily stood there for what seemed like a very long time and finally responded, 'I think I won't talk about being an eagle at school anymore.'

That was the day I hunted up my copy of Andersen's *The Ugly Duckling* and read to her about another creature who struggled with being different."

Historical Truth and Narrative Truth

According to those who study philosophy, there are two types of truth: historical truth and narrative truth (Ricoeur, 1983, 1985; Spence, 1982). Historical truth refers to the brute facts or data in an event. It is frequently very difficult to know the historical truth. More often, events are recorded in the form of what is called narrative truth. Narrative truth is a *reconstruction*, the product of its creator (the narrator) who describes events as *he or she* perceives them. The story of Emily contains both historical and narrative truth. If we were to ask, "What is the historical truth?" ("What are the facts?") in the preceding narrative, that would be difficult—perhaps impossible—to answer. After all, we have both Emily's and her mother's versions of events to sort through. Nevertheless, this simple story has been repeated to several groups of occupational therapy students. Each time it has been told it has been told a little differently. Sometimes the students hear that Emily is in "school," sometimes that she is in "preschool." Sometimes her words are, "I'm going to be a golden eagle," sometimes, she will be a "huge eagle." With each retelling, the students have been expected to believe, on faith perhaps, that it is a story based on historical truth. If liberties are taken with the historical truth, the story is still the same at its heart.

Comparing Clinical Stories with Case Reports

Ours is a book of stories that contain historical truth but most directly depict narrative truth. In a way, they are like folk tales, which may change in the retelling, but whose themes remain intact. Our clinical stories also are something like the case reports familiar in occupational therapy education and health care, but they are by no means as formal as most case reports, and they aspire toward a different goal. Before we begin our stories, we'd like to make a few comments about how case reports and clinical stories are similar or divergent in the way they use historical and narrative truth to teach.

To review, the case report in health care is a communication and reasoning tool which strives to organize the information therapists have about the individuals they serve. The case model of organizing data and planning treatment has a long history of use in the classroom and the conference room. The case report traditionally has provided a blend of historical fact and anecdotal or narrative information that could include client demographics; family, social, rehabilitation, and/or medical history; assessment data; intervention goals; significant marker events in the treatment course; evidence of change; and prognosis. Case reports usually emphasize historical facts, and often include measurable data. Rather than trying to stir the readers'/listeners' feelings, these reports are designed to help professionals stand back and reason with their intellect or to be objective. As Spence (1982) proposes, case reports may have a problem because they present only facts and facts don't always speak for themselves. Although historical data may appear objective, Schank (1994) describes them as "deceptive" because they give the "sense of knowing" without the "significance of knowing" (p. 32). Also, case facts often seem strung like different-sized beads that haven't been tied together. It is understandable, then, that many case reports are shaped by the biases (or "truths") of the narrator (case presenter) who reconstructs particular events. This includes selecting which details to emphasize and which to ignore, setting a stage or context for understanding the events, determining a chronology for how events will be presented, and, often, weaving in an interpretation of what really happened. Having been provided with case information, a reader or case conference participant might be asked to hypothesize about why events in treatment proceeded as they did, or to suggest solutions for as yet unresolved case problems. However, it is important to realize that once events have been reconstructed, they have moved outside of historical truth. One does not have an objective account of events, even if maintaining objectivity is a desired goal in the traditional case report. Although the readers'/listeners' task in reviewing a case is to stand outside and look on, in many case reports an unseen narrator leads them through the report, telling them what to notice and what it means.

Some case reports become more like stories powerfully driven by the narrator. As such, they represent a not-so-distant relative to the clinical stories that we present in this book.

Clinical Stories as Folk Tales

Clinical stories also have a long tradition, but one made in hallways and over cups of coffee. When therapists stop to tell about "what happened today" with a particular patient or client, they create these stories. Clients and family members have their own stories to tell as they share aloud "what happened today" from their point of view. In more recent occupational therapy literature (Clark, 1993; Fazio, 1992; Fine, 1993; Mattingly, 1991; Mattingly & Fleming, 1994; Peloquin, 1990), we encounter clinical stories that have been carefully crafted and used as a means to describe or enhance the experience of therapy.

Clinical stories, like case reports, crystallize thinking around events in therapy, and typically focus attention on a particular client or clients. Like case descriptions, these stories include a blend of historical and narrative truth. Unlike case reports, they often compromise historical fact, though we may, as Spence (1982) suggests, still come out wiser.

Like any good folk tale, clinical stories often have a moral or central message that represents the greater narrative truth that historical data can't capture. Clinical stories allow the narrator to illustrate rather than specify and often use evocative language rich in metaphor (Spence, 1982). Clinical stories, like folk tales, lead us to wonder "What will happen next?" as we follow the activities of individuals whom we expect to be somehow changed by the story's end. In looking at what brings about changes in the lives of their characters, clinical stories, like folk tales, are able to speak of human motives, values, desires, and disappointments (i.e., to all of the feelings that have no place among historical facts).

The stories in this book came about because each contributor was eager to tell about his or her experiences in therapy, and wanted to relate the truth as he or she saw it, and thereby create an experience the reader could understand and hopefully care about. Recounting stories of this kind is nestled in the belief that truth is subjective, or person-centered, and doesn't concern itself with the question of "Is this precisely what happened, or how it happened?" When we ask someone to write or tell a story, we in a sense say, "Be subjective. Put yourself into the story and show us how it was for you."

The Listener's Truth

Back to our would-be eagle, Emily. She, as many children, loved the story of the ugly duckling. When she first heard it she commented about the "poor baby duck," noting "how bad it must feel that no one will play with it." She talked about how she'd like to take it home and be its "mother." She took a step into the world of the duckling. She did so based on her own experience of the world, and her particular need to be nurtured and to nurture. Each time she listened to the story, she heard that story just a little differently than anyone who had ever heard it as she selected what to pay attention to and gave it meaning.

In much the same way, each clinical narrative in this book becomes the reader's story, your story, as you fit it into your personal beliefs, experiences, and picture of the world. Storytelling is only part of the process. The other part is story hearing.

Story Hearing—A New Paradigm for Learning

There has been a tradition in science, including the social sciences, to regard as absolute the claims based on empirical evidence or historical truth. In the past, therapists trying to use these facts to make practice decisions were admonished that to make the most of the information they had available, it was vital to keep their feelings separate from their intellect. For therapists working with clients or patients in the clinic, this meant not letting feelings get in the way of clear thinking. Even if therapists were to get close to their patients in day-to-day activities, when it came time to make treatment decisions it was important to stand back and be objective. The case presentation was a logical part of that tradition.

More recently, especially in the last decade, there has been what Ely and colleagues (1995) call a "paradigm shift," reflected in part by the renewed interest in qualitative (rather than quantitative) research in the social sciences, but evidenced throughout virtually all fields from law to philosophy, from medicine to physics (p. 3). It is a paradigm that embraces subjective rather than objective truth. In occupational therapy, it is supported by the work of Mattingly and Fleming (1994), who write that, in their practice, occupational therapists are concerned with the "lived body" and with "understanding people in terms of their daily practices, life histories, social relationships, and long-term projects, all of which give them a sense of meaning and a sense of personal identity" (pp. 64-65). In this newer way of looking at things, it is taken for granted that therapists cannot and should not try to keep feelings or values separate from their intellect in the effort to understand their clients' needs and make clinical judgments and practice decisions. Among the beliefs that this paradigm embraces are: (1) we as therapists will know the most about people (e.g., our clients and patients) when we understand their experiences, as much as possible, as they live or feel them, and (2) the way to do this is to own rather than disown our feelings and values, and to recognize these as partners, along with our intellect, in the process of understanding our clients and making practice decisions. Stories are well-suited to this newer paradigm for learning.

What You Will Find in This Book

The first 13 chapters in this book contain one or more stories told or written by an occupational therapist. The book's final chapter presents a personal account contributed by a client, Kevin, with additional comments from his spouse. In total, these stories describe therapeutic interactions among clients, therapists, family members, and other professionals within a milieu created by the helping community. Although emphasis is placed on the clients' and therapists' feelings and perceptions, we also examine issues relating to health care delivery criteria (e.g., probable duration of treatment and reimbursement). We learn how perceptions, feelings, and values integrate with knowledge, theoretical beliefs, and setting-specific expectations to bring about change and impact lives. Within these narratives, there are decisions to be made, often by the therapist, but also by the client or others. To the extent that each of you can place yourself in each story, these stories allow you to synthesize what you know and apply it to real situations.

Each chapter opens with Initial Comments in which the story's themes are identified and contextual information is provided to help the reader orient to the story. In many stories, the narrator refers to particular diagnoses or intervention strategies, or otherwise uses language associated with the narrator's frame of reference (also referred to as practice model). To ensure that the authors and reader have a shared understanding of clinically relevant material, we have summarized concepts which we feel to be especially important. However, we are not suggesting that this text substitute for others that provide a more in-depth presentation of didactic information. Rather, we see this book and other texts as companions. In our Initial Comments, we often alert the reader to crucial elements within the story, but we take care to avoid revealing the story's outcome.

Initial Comments are followed by the story itself. Some stories are brief vignettes, others are well developed. Each story has been given a title, usually the name of the story's main figure. Many of our contributing therapists are comfortable with being identified, while others prefer to remain anonymous. We have respected the wishes of each therapist. Those persons contributing stories were not selected for their expertise where a specialty area is depicted in the story. In fact, many levels of therapist expertise are represented. As authors, we included our own stories.

It was interesting to see, as the book took form, that similar themes were echoed throughout many of the stories. Stories were given to us either in writing or orally, and are presented as they were narrated, except as needed to protect confidentiality. In no instance did we ask any contributor to rewrite a story. The amount of detail, manner of presentation, and emphasis is unique to each narrative.

The ages of the clients around whose lives these stories revolve range from early adolescent to older adult. In several instances, the entire family can be viewed as a client. While most stories begin with a therapist-client interaction, in some stories the emphasis also is on the interaction of the therapist with other staff. The therapists contributing stories have a variety of roles in diverse settings. Some are full-time, others are temporary or per diem staff. They are employed in settings which include outpatient and inpatient hospital programs—psychiatric and nonpsychiatric, community programs and agencies, client homes, and skilled nursing and assisted-living facilities. Particular therapist roles identified include those of clinician, case manager, consultant, team member, registry therapist, and family liaison.

In each therapist's narrative, we learn about at least two individuals: the client and the therapist. The progress of each may create its own theme(s) and raise its own set of questions. We comment on both the therapist and the client in our text. Clients struggle to adapt to difficult circumstances and often loss; therapists strive to understand what their clients are going through, take into account the many circumstances that affect therapy, and make good decisions. Both want the client to have an improved quality of life. Themes that punctuate these narratives are related to control; loss and grief; motivation; internal and external resources and the climate for provision of service; fear, safety, and trust; the need to connect with others and to be heard and understood; rights and ethics;

dependence and independence; the significance of everyday skills and one's everyday environment; behavior management; and, above all, the need to live with dignity. However, the issues identified should not be viewed as the only important ones in the stories; readers and instructors may recognize other themes they will wish to explore.

In many of the stories, the narrator describes ambivalence regarding the decisions he or she or others made in the story. As therapists, we sometimes best remember those situations in which we have some lingering uncertainty. Often, too, these represent therapeutic experiences from which we can learn a great deal. We are reminded of the words of Langer (1994), who writes, "If I have no uncertainty about your always being right, no matter how important the issue may be, there is no reason to recognize how either of us might have changed. Certainty leads to mindlessness. Uncertainty, on the other hand, promotes mindfulness" (p. 46). We hope that through this text we stimulate mindfulness.

In our estimation, there are few, if any, instances where only one correct way to understand events, or only one appropriate course of action, exists in the scenarios depicted. We appreciate that our contributors have been willing to share their stories and doubts. Rather than criticizing or praising practice, we have tried to use Discussion Questions and our Impressions following the stories as a place to encourage flexible thinking, as we ask "How else might this (situation) have been viewed?" or "What might I have been done differently?" or "Why did this (strategy) seem to work so well?" We realize that stories may not depict ideal practice. As part of thinking about these stories, readers can begin to identify what constitutes sound practice and generate ideas about how practice might be improved.

The questions we have posed are multipurpose and vary in their difficulty level. Some questions can be answered with relative spontaneity, others might require that the reader consult additional sources. The questions relate to events in the story and bring the reader's attention to the many variables that influence the story's outcome. Readers may choose or be asked to answer some or all of the questions. Some questions ask about feelings depicted within and evoked by the story. Other questions ask readers to synthesize and apply knowledge (e.g., to identify theoretical assumptions evident within a story, identify specific precautions and resources applicable in the situation described, or suggest alternative approaches to problem solving).

We hope that there will be opportunities for faculty to facilitate small group discussion around the problem solving illustrated in the stories. We expect students to bring a variety of personal and professional experiences to their understanding of these stories. By responding to these questions within a peer discussion, students with diverse experiences can learn from each other.

Although the questions posed after each narrative are specific to that particular story, questions throughout the text in general ask the reader to empathize with clients and therapists, relate knowledge and theoretical perspectives to the events of the story, identify beliefs, form opinions, and hypothesize about what to do in similar circumstances. Yet our questions are only a skeleton. Instructors may want to add or substitute their own, or ask students to generate questions. Most scenarios present multiple and diverse concerns that need to be addressed. Our particular emphasis has been on the emotional and psychosocial side, but in concern for the whole person-in-the-environment. Individual instructors may give the material a different emphasis, or use it as a point of departure for independent learning experiences.

Discussion Questions are followed by our commentary. This section, Impressions, may summarize our experiences in similar therapy situations. Many of the stories written by our contributors prompted us to recall our own experiences in practice. We refer to these to provide additional contexts in which the story's theme or key issues arise, and thereby help emphasize the breadth of the issue and the many possibilities one has in responding.

In Impressions, we respond with relative freedom to the events and issues that were presented in each story, much as we might in a classroom discussion. In this section, we reflect on the story's course and on how clients have changed or therapists have been affected. We highlight therapeutic principles and practices and may suggest alternative ways of approaching specific challenges depicted in the story. We share our own reactions, including our feelings about the events within the story, and identify what we have learned. If what each reader sees in every story filters through his or her personal lenses, nowhere is that more apparent than in the impressions that we as authors share. The reader will find that different issues and content move each of us in many instances. Our impressions are not value-free; our biases are articulated openly. We expect that as you read and dialogue with your instructor and peers, you also will be drawn to diverse themes and will become more aware of your own values and beliefs, which may stand in sharp contrast to ours.

Using This Text to Enhance Clinical Reasoning Skills

Both of us, as authors, have had and continue to have many roles and responsibilities within occupational therapy practice and education, from writing to instructing to continued daily practice. The common thread through our experiences has been teaching—teaching here characterized as both fun and hard work. Our goal has been to write a text that shows how theory, knowledge, philosophy, individual personalities, and those myriad "somethings" that make each situation different from every other come together to comprise the real world of occupational therapy practice. We believe this is depicted through these stories, and within the context of these stories students can get a sense of how alive psychosocial interaction in practice really is. We have added questions and our comments to provide tools for helping students participate in clinical reasoning. We use language that we hope puts the reader at ease and helps engender a comfortable feeling, and invites inquiry and involvement with the material.

The challenge in health care is largely to use one's knowledge and thinking to solve problems effectively. As discussed previously, problem solving in occupational therapy may begin with the gathering of extensive case information, such as that provided in medical and social histories and formal occupational therapy interviews and assessment. However, therapists do not always have this traditional case information available when they commence intervention. Time allowed for occupational therapy may be limited, and interdisciplinary meetings may be relatively infrequent. Whether starting therapy with a new client, or working with a client over an extended period, therapists often need to draw upon what they know, synthesize information, make decisions, and respond quickly. This requires considerable problem solving, and challenges both the novice and the experienced therapist.

The literature (Mattingly & Fleming, 1994; Royeen, 1995; VanLeit, 1995) and our own observations tell us that, when problem solving, therapists use different types of clinical reasoning to pull together knowledge, specific skills, and strategies within practice. Often, experienced therapists can quickly call upon previous similar experiences to generate alternatives in responding to the daily problems of clinical practice. The experienced therapist can come up with many ways to resolve a problem or complete a task, and can, as needed, step back and evaluate how effective his or her actions have been (Ross, 1989; Roth, 1989).

On the other hand, students and beginning practitioners usually do not have an extensive repertoire of clinical experiences to draw upon as they make decisions. They more often make decisions based on rules and principles learned in school, and they may or may not take into full account the many variables particular to an individual client's needs. These beginners may have only one or a limited number of familiar ways to approach and solve a clinical problem.

Each of our stories illustrates the process or outcome of clinical reasoning. Each also provides an opportunity to practice clinical reasoning. Our hope is that you can put yourself in the stories and move around, so to speak, to imagine how the individuals might have viewed events and how they might have felt; then, discover and discuss how you might use what you know, what you believe, and what you feel in order to reason and respond in the situations described.

The Benefits of Story Sharing

Therapists, it seems, love to tell stories about their patients or clients, just as patients and family members want their stories heard. Telling stories can be a way of making sense of seemingly disparate events; it can be an avenue to think out loud about "What do I do next?" It can be a means for wrapping up or getting closure, or a way of connecting with other people and seeing that "We've all had this happen." In their stories, therapists seek validation as they ask their colleagues, "Does it sound like what I did was okay?" Stories can be a door to healing and a way to give words to our anger or our hope. Stories undoubtedly can be a vehicle for clinical reasoning. Most of all, stories provide a means to keep our special experiences alive.

References

Clark, F. (1993). Occupation imbedded in real life: Interweaving occupational science and occupational therapy. *American Journal of Occupational Therapy, 47,* 1067-1077.

Ely, M., Anzul, M., Friedman, T., Garner, D., & Steinmetz, A.M. (1995). *Doing qualitative research: Circles within circles.* Bristol, PA: Falmer Press (Taylor and Francis).

Fazio, L. (1992). Tell me a story: The therapeutic metaphor in the practice of pediatric occupational therapy. *American Journal of Occupational Therapy, 46,* 1067-1077.

Fine, S. (1993). Interaction between psychological variables and cognitive function. In C.B. Royeen (Ed.), *AOTA self-study series: Cognitive rehabilitation.* Rockville, MD: American Occupational Therapy Association.

Langer, E. (1994). The illusion of calculated decisions. In R.C. Schank and E. Langer (Eds.), *Beliefs, reasoning, and decision making: Psycho-logic in honor of Bob Abelson.* Hillsdale, NJ: Lawrence Erlbaum.

Mattingly, C. (1991). The narrative nature of clinical reasoning. *American Journal of Occupational Therapy, 45,* 998-1005.

Mattingly, C., & Fleming, M. (1994). *Clinical reasoning: Forms of inquiry in a therapeutic practice.* Philadelphia: F.A. Davis.

Peloquin, S. (1990). The patient-therapist relationship in occupational therapy: Understanding visions and images. *American Journal of Occupational Therapy, 44,* 13-21.

Ricoeur, P. (1983). *Time and narrative* (K. McLaughline & D. Pellauer, Trans.). (Vol. 3). Chicago: University of Chicago Press.

Ricoeur, P. (1985). *Reality of the historical past.* Milwaukee, WI: Marquette University Press.

Ross, D.A. (1989, March-April). First steps in developing a reflective approach. *Journal of Teacher Education,* 22-30.

Roth, D.A. (1989, March-April). Preparing the reflective practitioner: Transforming the apprentice through the dialectic. *Journal of Teacher Education,* 31-35.

Royeen, C.R. (1995). A problem-based learning curriculum for occupational therapy education. *American Journal of Occupational Therapy, 49,* 338-346.

Schank, R.C. (1994). Goal-based scenarios. In R.C. Schank and E. Langer (Eds.), *Beliefs, reasoning, and decision making: Psycho-logic in honor of Bob Abelson.* Hillsdale, NJ: Lawrence Erlbaum.

Spence, D. (1982). *Narrative truth and historical truth: Meaning and interpretation in psychoanalysis.* New York: Norton.

VanLeit, B. (1995). Using the case method to develop clinical reasoning skills in problem-based learning. *American Journal of Occupational Therapy, 49,* 349-353.

CHAPTER 1

Therapeutic Relationship

KEY TOPICS

- Humanism
- Client-centered occupational therapy
- Therapeutic relationship
- Difficult clients
- Paranoia
- Confrontation
- Control
- Patient rights
- Caregiver rights
- Responding to attention-seeking behavior

Initial Comments

Struggling with physical and psychological challenges can bring into sharp focus concerns that our clients have around their own abilities, and around their feelings that they have too little say or even no control over the events of their daily lives. For some people, this results in being inflexible or demanding; for others, it can lead to a wish to give up choices and let someone else be in charge. One of occupational therapy's most significant contributions is providing opportunities for individuals to experience themselves as effective or empowered. At the same time, resumption of meaningful occupation often necessitates a reappraisal of one's own limits.

This and the next chapter share several themes, including the need of the central persons to exert control in their lives while managing limitations. Jane, the client in this story, appears to have difficulty establishing a comfortable give-and-take relationship with those around her. She alternately makes demands on people and creates barriers between herself and others.

If Jane is to become successfully engaged in therapy, it will be a priority that the occupational therapist deal with this dimension of Jane's behavior. Before her initial visit, the occupational therapist sent to see Jane in her home has been apprised that Jane is a difficult client. This therapist describes her own approach as "client-centered," referring to an implementation in practice of humanistic-existential tenets (Bruce & Borg, 1993). The narrative that follows, plus several other stories in this book, make particular reference to humanistic ideology. Because humanistic beliefs are so central to the practice of occupational therapy and are evidenced throughout the text, and in order to help you place yourself in this story, we begin by highlighting what is meant by the terms "humanism" and "client-centered" in occupational therapy.

Humanistic Philosophy in Occupational Therapy

The humanistic-existential roots of the profession go back to such early writers as Meyer (1922), Slagle (1922), and Dunton (1919), and have been eloquently reaffirmed in the professional literature from the 1960s through the present day (Baum, 1980; Devereaux, 1984; Gilfoyle, 1980; Law, Baptiste, & Mills, 1995; Mattingly & Fleming, 1994; Peloquin, 1990; Yerxa, 1967, 1978, 1991). These occupational therapists emphasize that occupational therapy has a humanistic foundation built on the belief that the people served (clients) are unique and valuable individuals, that each client is the real expert on his or her life, and that in the context of a therapeutic relationship, the client can take an active role in directing the course of his or her own therapy. In Canada in 1983, occupational therapists as a national group articulated and endorsed what they referred to as a model of "client-centered practice" based upon a marriage of occupational therapy concepts and humanistic-existential tenets (Canadian Association of Occupational Therapists and Department of National Health and Welfare, 1983). This model continues to act as a common denominator for practice in Canada (Law et al., 1995).

Nature of the Person in Humanism

According to humanistic theory, the person is essentially positive, possessing the ability for self-awareness and having the responsibility for shaping his or her own life. As described by such humanistic writers as May (1950, 1953, 1969, 1975), Rogers (1951, 1961), Moustakas (1961), and Maslow (1968) in psychology, and those previously cited in occupational therapy, each individual experiences an innate striving toward health, wholeness, and greater experience. Therefore, as therapists we do not have to motivate people to "get well" or to develop their abilities within occupation; that motivation is believed to exist in each of us. Also suggested is an innate and healthy need for autonomy, a need to take charge of one's own life-path. That is not to say that we do not all have to negotiate limitations in our abilities and resources.

Phenomenology

According to this framework, each person lives in his or her own perceptual or phenomenological world. Psychologist Arthur Combs (1972) writes, "...the individual's behavior is seen as the direct consequence, not of the fact or stimulus with which he (or she) is confronted, but of the meaning of events in his (or her) peculiar economy" (p. 118). Restated, it's not just what each person faces daily, it's how he (or she) perceives it. If, for instance, a patient or client is offered a chance to live independently, or to learn a new computer skill, but thinks to himself or herself, "I could never do that," then in a sense the choice doesn't really exist. Similarly, a family that doesn't perceive itself as able to cope with a member who has a disability may sabotage efforts to bring its family member home, because family members can't imagine how the arrangement could ever work out.

People, too, gain a picture of themselves within this perceptual world, including who they are (both positive and negative) and what they can and cannot do. People tend to block out, deny, or distort any information that contradicts that image. One way to describe what happens is that people develop blind spots. There are things about themselves that others can see, but they cannot. Even when given feedback, individuals may be unable to use that information effectively.

Meaningfulness and Context

The individual needs to see the self in a consistent way and to perceive the relevance of experience. In a real sense, the participant in therapy must be able to say about his or her experience, "I am doing this because it is important to me." This depends on one's ability to fit an experience into a larger picture. For occupational therapists, this suggests that our clients must understand how the activities or occupations in therapy make a meaningful fit within the context of their everyday lives. Clients' values as imbued in their "roles, interests, environments, and culture" anchor client-centered practice (Law et al., 1995, p. 252).

Function

With a humanistic orientation, optimum function exists when the person experiences relative comfort with himself or herself, is open to experience, is guided by his or her own beliefs and values, and uses existing skills and abilities to the fullest degree to perform valued life tasks, while behaving in a manner that respects the rights and needs of others.

Therapeutic Relationship at the Heart of Intervention

Psychologist and author Carl Rogers (1951) introduced the concept of client-centered therapy to describe a helping relationship in which the therapist strives to understand the meaning of a client's experiences from the client's perspective. Rather than judge this other person, the therapist wants to be able to understand what it's like to be in this person's shoes. The course of therapy is set by what the client values, what activities are meaningful, and what therapeutic goals the client would like to achieve. Assessment is individualized accordingly as the therapist gathers information about what is important to the client. Perhaps the single best client-centered assessment tool is the open-ended question, or request to "Tell me about your concerns."

Emphasis is placed on the therapist's role in the relationship. Clients are believed most likely to flourish within a relationship where the therapist is genuine, communicates caring and respect, and abides by the belief that the client has much wisdom about what he or she needs to accomplish in therapy.

The therapeutic relationship becomes one of collaboration or partnership, where the therapist uses his or her expertise to identify the means to achieve desired goals. As articulated by Law et al. (1995), the client-centered model is one of "enablement" in which "therapists work with clients to enable them to achieve occupational therapy goals that they have set for themselves" (p. 252). The client and therapist can work together to achieve what neither could achieve alone (Law et al., 1995, p. 252).

Changing Perceptions, Expanding Possibilities

According to this model, the success of intervention will depend not on therapists' knowledge or techniques or what therapists teach per se, but on "the degree to which (we) understand the perceptual worlds of those (we) seek to work with and become skillful in helping others to change their perceptions of themselves and their surroundings" (Combs, 1972, p. 123). This is because people tend to take from therapy that which fits their self-image and their understanding of the world around them.

The individual is most able to use his or her potential within occupation and to be open to change in the context of the therapeutic relationship when he or she feels accepted and acceptable. Client-centered therapists don't demand that a person be all he or she can be, nor insist that he or she learn, rather, they create a context that allows this to happen.

Using Occupation

Therapeutic activities can include any that increase knowledge and understanding, and move the client toward meeting occupational goals.

Within mental health occupational therapy practice, activities originating from humanism-existentialism are aimed primarily at increasing insight and self-awareness. These include values clarification activities, body awareness and relaxation experiences, journaling, storytelling, and gestalt art experiences. Although these activities may be used more frequently in psychosocial occupational therapy settings, they may be adapted for other rehabilitation settings in which they are offered to people who have experienced trauma and are coping with long-term disability (e.g., people with brain or spinal cord injury) (Borg & Bruce, 1991; Dougherty & Radomski, 1987). However, virtually any activity in any setting can enhance or be adapted toward the goals of client-centered practice. Client-centered occupation helps the client accomplish what he or she values.

What Client-Centered Can Mean in Everyday Intervention

More broadly, client-centered means putting the client's needs first. Therapists make decisions every day that reflect their concern for the client's values (e.g., their understanding that clients may be self-conscious about their bodies or performance) or their realization that living with disabilities can be very stressful. Being client-centered includes scheduling intervention at times that fit the needs of the client and allowing time for rest if the client desires. Being client-centered means not pushing clients to finish because we have someone else we need to see, and being sensitive to a person's wish for privacy when assisting with showering or dressing. Client-centered language is that which clients can understand. Therapists are client-centered when they help clients avoid embarrassment about unavoidable body odors or when unexpected incontinence brings attention to them. Sometimes clients express their appreciation for this humanistic approach simply by saying, "Thank you for your kindness."

An Instance of Views at Odds

This story is one in which each of the individuals in the story perceives shared events and their meanings differently. As noted earlier, an angry confrontation occurs in the story, but there are actually several opportunities for constructive confrontation. In the humanistic usage, confrontation refers to a process by which we bring information to an individual's attention that lay outside of his or her awareness. Confrontation is not viewed as an angry or negative act, as develops in this story, but as a way of letting a person know how events may look different to different people. If confrontational material is presented (or perceived) as a criticism or an attack, then, in humanistic thinking, we would expect the individual to behave defensively or reject the information. Since confrontation is so significant in this story, we would like you to pay particular attention to how it was and how it might have been handled.

The Impact of Paranoid Disorder

The option of using confrontative techniques is drawn into question when the narrating therapist introduces the possibility that the client has or has had a paranoid disorder. Paranoid disorders are striking instances of problems with trust and closeness, and they impose the potential for a skewed interpretation of events. With paranoid disorders, a therapeutic relationship may be especially hard to achieve.

Without applying any diagnostic labels, we can add to our contextual understanding by reviewing some of the classical signs associated with paranoid thinking. *Kaplan and Sadock's Synopsis of Psychiatry* (7th ed.) (Kaplan, Sadock, & Grebb, 1994) discusses paranoid thinking as displayed in paranoid personality disorder. It is described as an "unwarranted tendency...to interpret other people's actions as deliberately demeaning or threatening" and having a distrust of people in general. People who tend toward paranoia "refuse responsibility for their own feelings and assign responsibility to others" and are "often hostile, irritable, and angry." Examples in everyday terms include the "bigot," "injustice collector," and "litigious crank" (Kaplan et al., 1994, p. 734). According to the *Diagnostic and Statistical Manual of Mental Disorders* (4th ed.) ([*DSM-IV*] American Psychiatric Association, 1994), the person who tends toward paranoid thinking often bears "grudges" or is "unforgiving of insults or slights," and is "easily slighted and quick to react with anger or to counterattack" (Kaplan et al., 1994, p. 734). But the *DSM-IV* includes an important qualifier when it suggests that the person demonstrating paranoid thinking "suspects *without sufficient basis* that others are exploiting, harming, or deceiving him or her" (emphasis ours) (Kaplan et al., 1994, p. 734).

When patients or clients tend toward mistrust and seem especially irritable, and, as occurs in our first story, are abrasive, care providers may begin to dismiss client complaints or legitimate requests as unreasonable without giving them adequate attention. However, this can occur any time patients or clients question the treatment they are receiving. No one likes to hear that they're not doing a good job, and even with all the best intentions, staff can have tunnel vision and block out feedback that is disconcerting.

Applying a label such as "paranoid" runs contrary to basic humanistic ideology, as it is a box that tends to limit rather than expand possibilities for human experience. However, the client has indicated to the therapist that she feels mistreated. For occupational therapists in this situation, it is especially important to be straightforward with clients, share information openly, and enable appropriate involvement in the decision-making process, which is consistent with both the approach recommended for responding to paranoid thought disorder (Kaplan et al., 1994, p. 735) and with client-centered occupational therapy.

"Jane" Narrated by Barbara Borg, MA, OTR

You knew the minute you walked into her apartment that she was artistic and paid attention to detail. Everything was just so. Each object had been carefully chosen and placed to carry the eye around a striking and tasteful room. The surprise was in how much of the room's contents Jane said she had made herself: the paintings, the pillows, some vases, even the bedspread. This woman was a former art teacher who stated that years earlier she had "thought about" being an occupational therapist. With all its angles, the room had somewhat of a masculine feel, but was softened by the many pictures of her children and their children, all of whom lived out-of-state. It was only after I had come to know her better that she told me that she had been married for a short time, and that her husband took his own life by shooting himself in the head.

For as much as one felt drawn to the room, its lone occupant tried to keep visitors at a distance. Jane was a 56-year-old woman who, being tall and about 40 pounds overweight with a rather ruddy complexion, appeared robust. However, she had severe chronic obstructive pulmonary disease (COPD), and postponed using the bathroom and eating because both demanded breath she couldn't find. She was on three liters of continuous oxygen, and on many days she had to pause between each word just to speak.

She also had fibromyalgia, a disease that causes muscle pain in what is believed to be an autoimmune reaction. Jane let everyone know that she was in near-constant pain. Sometimes she would holler out unexpectedly and people in the room would jump, startled and frightened by her shouting. More than once the resident staff where she lived called an ambulance, afraid that she was in some kind of imminent danger. Eventually they began to ignore her crying and yelling, apparently assuming that she was just looking for attention.

The first time I phoned Jane to set up an appointment, I called knowing that she had refused the services of several care providers who had been sent to her home. She allowed that I might come, but at the conclusion of my first visit, she said, "I don't know what you can do for me...You don't need to come back." On a hunch, I responded that I'd like to give her a bit of time to think about that and indicated I'd return on the following "Wednesday afternoon at 4:00." I told her that I'd ring her buzzer and she'd have the choice then of whether or not to let me in. After that, she seemed anxious to have me visit, and over the next 3 weeks called the office several times to request that I come for an extra visit or simply give her a call.

Because her shortness of breath made it difficult to perform the most basic tasks, I wanted to determine if she knew and could use pursed lip, diaphragmatic breathing. I figured that if she knew the basics of this technique, we could work on incorporating it into her daily routines. I demonstrated the technique, and explained that it might also help her to relax when she felt especially stressed or felt her pain was worsening. She responded by telling me that she had been shown these techniques before but had "never gotten the hang of them." We talked about the advantage of integrating deep, cleansing breaths into brief periods of activity, principles of energy conservation, and the possible benefits of taking time out during the day to lie down and use deep breathing as a kind of meditative tool. She agreed she would again try to learn these techniques. When I asked what she hoped to accomplish in therapy, she responded that her goals included being able to breathe well enough to leave her apartment complex for brief periods and to manage the pain of her fibromyalgia better. Resident staff had told me that she was "impossible" to get along with, and she told me that she thought the staff were rude, that they often talked about her, and that they ignored her. So it seemed an equally important therapy goal would be to help Jane and those in her daily life better understand each other and meet each other's needs.

I found some literature that suggested keeping muscles moving through simple, low-stress physical activity to manage fibromyalgia, and we discussed the possibility of getting her involved in a therapeutic aquatic program at a nearby rehabilitation center. The literature also suggested that stress contributed to the exacerbation of pain.

Weeks 2-4

My efforts at teaching diaphragmatic breathing were proving only marginally successful. Jane refused to sit up straight or lie flat to open her airways during diaphragmatic breathing because her chest muscles "hurt," and she persisted in a semi-slumped posture. She also had difficulty maintaining slow, pursed-lip expiration. She sometimes could do it if I was standing by her bed cuing her, but I had to be careful not to stand too close to her. On one occasion, when I was demonstrating proper exhalation, she barked, "Back away! You're blowing on me." After a few attempts, she said flatly that she would not attempt to use this breathing technique in my absence because it was "too damn confusing." The general tenor of my response to Jane—when she refused to sit up straight and said she wouldn't practice deep breathing on her own—was that I understood that this way of breathing often felt very unnatural in the beginning, but that for it to work best, it should be practiced correctly. I told her that the choice was hers, and that I wasn't asking for any promises she wouldn't keep. Then I suggested that each day she might want to try a few cleansing breaths on her own and gradually become more accustomed to how that feels. During one of my visits, we spent most of the hour assessing her shower routine while I recommended adaptations that would conserve strength and energy. On another occasion, we engaged in a similar process around dressing and grooming.

I continued to spend the first 15 minutes or so of our sessions cuing her on the deep breathing pattern and helping her to reposition. After several sessions, I incorporated some simple visual imagery into these instructions. I also spent considerable time trying to get to know her better and build rapport.

Two incidents underscored the problems Jane had with relating interpersonally. In my second week of seeing her, I had scheduled a visit to coincide with her lunchtime so I could observe her eating. She wasn't able to go to the common dining room, so a teenage employee delivered lunch to her room. Lunch included a baked potato but lacked the sour cream Jane had requested. "How can I eat this crap?" she screeched at the befuddled high-schooler, and insisted the potato be taken back to the kitchen. In between labored breaths, she cursed the food, the staff, and life in general.

About a week later, I knocked at her door and Jane was standing right there, ready to let me in. She was eager to tell me about something that had happened the day before. She related that her visiting nurse had stopped by, apparently to check her vital signs. The nurse had started to unbutton Jane's blouse in order to listen to her heart and lungs with a stethoscope. The nurse had apparently startled Jane, who pulled away and yelled at her, "What are you doing?" Jane refused to let the nurse proceed. The two got into a shouting match, with the nurse finally screaming at Jane, "You are a horrid lady and you need to be in a mental hospital." I later learned that Jane had been in a mental hospital many years earlier. Around the time her husband had died, she was in treatment for problems relating to being "suicidal" and "paranoid." I was able to talk with her visiting nurse who agreed that the events had occurred pretty much as Jane described. The nurse added, "I just lost it...I can't stand that woman." I knew the nurse well and was very surprised that she could get this upset and respond as she had. It led me to think about how successfully Jane could get under others' skin. This nurse asked to be relieved of her responsibility for Jane, and resigned from the agency not too long after this incident.

One of the most difficult tasks for me was feeling clear on whether or not others actually mistreated Jane. During each visit, she described instances in which she felt she had been treated unfairly or rudely. One of the things that struck me was how circumscribed her world had become—it was a world that revolved around the visits of therapists and nurses. Being client-centered from way back, I mostly listened to her concerns and empathized. I tried to withhold judgment, believing that whatever she was telling me was reality as far as she had perceived it. Then I tried to help her to decenter—to stand back and consider what others might have been feeling, or to try and put herself in their place. In my estimation, I did this very gently and with much tentativeness in my voice, allowing her to either validate or dispute my observations. I felt that if she saw me as critical of her, she'd put up a wall against anything I said. Her interaction with the visiting nurse was corroborated, but most everyday events were not. There were, I felt, times when resident staff did the least possible for her because they so disliked her. I was able to observe a few occasions when she had what seemed like legitimate requests or concerns, and staff paid little attention, regarding them as complaints to be ignored. Was she paranoid and suspicious of others' intentions? Probably. Was she out of touch with reality? I didn't know. People didn't like her and she knew it, yet she surely helped create and perpetuate that state of affairs with her considerable complaining and shouting at staff. On the flip side, when I was with her I sensed that what she wanted was our time and positive attention. She was very articulate and was often very engaging. She liked to talk about politics and her family, and at times she had quite a sense of humor, albeit dry. But neither the resident nor treatment staff seemed to know this about her, and they certainly didn't give her the extra time or hugs that seemed lavished on other clients to help smooth over rough spots when problems arose with them.

The facility where Jane lived did not have to put up with her temper or irritability because there was a long waiting list of people wanting to live there. No particular event that I knew of precipitated this, but one day I went to see her and she said she was told she had to move. Her new residence had in-house therapists, so my intervention terminated. I visited her once after that and her COPD had worsened. I felt that she did not have much longer to live.

Discussion Questions

1. In what way does the narrator's perception of this client seem different from the visiting nurse's? Speculate on the reasons for this difference in perception.

2. How do you think you would feel working with this client?
3. What kinds of situations with or behaviors in another tend to "push your buttons"? How do you generally respond? Is this the same for you at work or school as in social situations?
4. How might you avoid problems if you anticipate that an individual may be difficult in therapy?
5. If you work or have worked in an intervention setting, what support is or was available for you to manage the behavior of difficult clients?
6. One occasion when the therapist might have confronted Jane regarding the impact of her behavior was when Jane yelled at the high-schooler serving lunch. Do you think the therapist should have intervened? If so, describe a strategy that the therapist could have used to respond to Jane. If not, why not?
7. When Jane refused to sit upright as shown and stated that she would not practice deep breathing outside the therapy hour, the therapist could have pointed out to Jane that her behavior seemed resistive to therapy. It would have been consistent with the protocol of the agency employing the therapist to terminate treatment. Discuss whether or not you think Jane should have been confronted and/or treatment terminated if she continued to resist doing the breathing exercises properly.
   a. Suggest alternative ways that the principles of deep breathing might be taught.
   b. If you were Jane, why might you resist this technique?
8. Have you ever witnessed unequal treatment of patients or clients? Was favor given to one person more than another, even when practice standards were met?
   a. What do you suppose contributed to this in terms of client behaviors, staff needs, environmental or situational demands, and resources?
   b. What feelings did this stir in you?
9. What are your options if a patient or client tells you that a treatment staff member has treated him or her disrespectfully?
   a. Are you aware of specific protocols that have been established to respond in such a situation in an agency where you have been employed or have observed?
10. Put yourself in Jane's place, and think about what the nurse in this situation might have done to help you feel more at ease.
11. Assume you are Jane's therapist. How could you have helped Jane learn to effectively articulate her needs in this kind of situation?
12. Put yourself in the nurse's place. What might you have been feeling when you were screamed at for doing what may have seemed like a routine part of your job?
    a. What may have contributed to the initial lack of sensitivity in this particular situation?

13. The therapist in this story applied principles closely identified with humanism and client-centered practice. Cite particular statements made by the narrator and actions taken that exemplify client-centered philosophy or practice.
14. Critique the selection and use of therapeutic activities. Are there others you might have tried?
15. Are there any other issues in this story that you feel might have warranted further attention? What are they?

Impressions

BB: Jane was my client and I have shared this account with my students. I use it to illustrate how the client-centered model can frame the way a client is perceived and decisions are made. As I reread this, I notice that it is a story about distance and boundaries.

I enjoyed her and she clearly wanted me to visit, but Jane could tolerate just so much closeness. An event that characterizes the story, for me, is when Jane tells me, "Back away! You're blowing on me." It seems reasonable to conclude that establishing a sound therapeutic relationship is a logical place to begin with Jane, and that I'd have to allow Jane her distance. I wouldn't expect Jane, who was wary and seemed to need to feel in control, to jump right into therapy or to make changes very quickly. It follows that unless Jane trusted me as her therapist and believed that therapeutic activities had the potential to help her, she wasn't likely to participate in therapy and therapy wouldn't help increase function. In terms of trying to give her feedback about her abrasive behavior and trying to help her decenter, as I describe, it appears especially vital that Jane feel safe with me.

Kaplan et al., who offer a psychodynamic perspective, provide a slightly different view on how best to respond to paranoid thinking. They say that mistrustful patients may become frightened if "they feel that those trying to help them are weak and helpless" (Kaplan et al., 1994, p. 735). Maybe Jane would have felt safer and cooperated more fully if I had been more directive with her. Jane might have perceived me as ineffectual in that I offered tentative interpretations of events and allowed her a good deal of control. We can only speculate.

Thinking about the evolution of this story from the viewpoint of other frames of reference in occupational therapy, I assume that the behaviorally oriented therapist may look at the encounter with Jane differently, and might ask, "What behaviors are you rewarding?" From that perspective, we can wonder if I was paying off Jane's resistive behaviors.

The client-centered stance taken in this story fits well with the psychoeducational model. Using psychoeducational principles to improve performance, we can help empower our clients by giving them information. I was doing that in teaching Jane about deep breathing and about energy conservation. Another aspect of that, it seems, could have centered on giving Jane more information about both her COPD and her fibromyalgia. Both the nurse and I could have collaborated more in that respect. One way this might have been enhanced would have been through her involvement in support groups, had she been in agreement.

One reason that I continue to have unsettled feelings about Jane and her story is that I felt that staff avoided her. I was concerned that even if her obvious physical needs were met, many less obvious needs were not. Granted, Jane pushes people away, or at least gives mixed messages. From the humanistic perspective, we could say that Jane behaves in a manner that affirms the negative picture others have of her and that she holds of herself.

MAB: There are several themes at work here. These center largely on the influence of the environment in which therapy occurs with Jane.

Although I cannot condone the nurse's behavior—her quick-paced movement to unbutton Jane's blouse and her angry response to Jane—I can understand how it might occur. As I have worked in various environments in the community and health care system, I have noted that staff members are pressured for productivity and efficiency. They must perform procedures quickly and then move to their next responsibility. This may interfere with humanistic practice. Or, when the care provider is fatigued and working under stress with a difficult client, he or she may not have the necessary energy or personal resources for client-centered problem solving. The focus becomes task accomplishment.

I agree that Jane's appearance and personality could impact her care. I sometimes feel that some patients are avoided—those who are difficult (e.g., angry or demanding) or who complain—especially if staff feel that there is no way to satisfy them. However, I feel that the problem goes beyond the patient-staff member interaction. Other care system issues need to be addressed. As care systems downsize, available resources for staff members may diminish. There may be, for instance, fewer opportunities to get support and problem solve through team planning meetings, there may be fewer educational programs for caregivers at all levels, and there may be less support (formal and informal) for working with difficult clients and patients.

Another system element that would affect occupational therapy intervention is the pressure from third-party payers to demonstrate and document change in function. This pressure does not always allow for the individual client to recover and progress at his or her own rate, particularly those persons with multiple, long-term, or chronic problems.

Staff may label patient, client, or student behavior as "attention seeking." This was typically expressed with a negative connotation, the implication being that the staff should avoid giving attention to the individual until he or she could ask for it more "appropriately." However, there was usually little or no role modeling of appropriate behavior, and the patient-staff struggle continued. I've worked and observed in some settings where behavior modification programs have been tried by treatment teams with varied success. I am usually not the one to recommend these strategies, but I have cooperated in their implementation to the best of my ability. I found that patients sometimes interpreted their treatment in these programs as being "disliked," or even "abused," by staff. I am more comfortable with cognitive behavior approaches for managing behavior.

Cognitive behavioral theory suggests that we use patient discussion and education as well as behavior modeling and management strategies. I prefer this approach with most age groups and disabilities. I find it much more effective, although perhaps I'm more comfortable with the theoretical principles. I also feel that cognitive behavioral orientation is compatible with humanistic perspectives.

From my humanistic or client-centered orientation, I assume that there must be a reason an individual is seeking attention. I may ask a person for clarification about what he or she needs, or I may try to put myself into his or her shoes—I have found both useful. As I empathize, I am reminded of my own need for attention when I'm not feeling well, or when I'm away from home and out of my familiar surroundings. And I think about how a quick "hello" from a neighbor, or even being greeted by a pet, can meet the need for attention. Sometimes something as simple as a good, hot cup of coffee can fill a void. Bringing a client a hot cup of coffee often goes a long way toward meeting their needs and limits further attention-seeking behavior.

References

American Psychiatric Association. (1994). *Diagnostic and statistical manual of mental disorders* (4th ed.). Washington, DC: Author.

Baum, C. (1980). Occupational therapists put care in the health system. *American Journal of Occupational Therapy, 34,* 505-516.

Borg, B., & Bruce, M.A. (1991). *The group system: The therapeutic activity group in occupational therapy.* Thorofare, NJ: SLACK Inc.

Bruce, M.A., & Borg, B. (1993). *Psychosocial occupational therapy: Frames of reference for intervention.* Thorofare, NJ: SLACK Inc.

Canadian Association of Occupational Therapists and Department of National Health and Welfare. (1983). *Guidelines for the client-centered practice of occupational therapy* (H39-33/1983E). Ottawa, Ontario, Canada: Department of National Health and Welfare.

Combs, A. (1972). Some basic concepts in perceptual psychology. In D.L. Avilla, A.W. Combs, & W.W. Purkey (Eds.), *The helping relationship sourcebook* (pp. 117-126). Boston: Allyn and Bacon.

Devereaux, E. (1984). Occupational therapy's challenge: The caring relationship. *American Journal of Occupational Therapy, 38,* 791-798.

Dougherty, P.M., & Radomski, M.V. (1987). *The cognitive rehabilitation workbook: A systematic approach to improving independent living skills in brain injured adults.* Rockville, MD: Aspen Publications.

Dunton, W. (1919). *Reconstruction therapy.* Philadelphia, W.B. Saunders.

Gilfoyle, E. (1980). Caring: A philosophy for practice. *American Journal of Occupational Therapy, 34,* 517-521.

Kaplan, H., Sadock, B., & Grebb, J. (1994). *Kaplan and Sadock's synopsis of psychiatry* (7th ed.). Baltimore: Williams & Wilkins.

Law, M., Baptiste, S., & Mills, J. (1995). Client-centered practice: What does it mean and does it make a difference? *Canadian Journal of Occupational Therapy, 62,* 250-257.

Maslow, A. (1968). *Toward a psychology of being* (Rev. ed.). New York: Van Nostrand.

Mattingly, C., & Fleming, M.H. (1994). *Clinical reasoning: Forms of inquiry in a therapeutic practice.* Philadelphia: F.A. Davis.

May, R. (1950). *The meaning of anxiety.* New York: Ronald Press.

May, R. (1953). *Man's search for himself.* New York: Norton.

May, R. (1969). *Love and will.* New York: Norton.

May, R. (1975). *The courage to create.* New York: Norton.

Meyer, A. (1922). The philosophy of occupational therapy. *Archives of Occupational Therapy, 1,* 1-10.

Moustakas, C. (1961). *Loneliness.* Englewood Cliffs, NJ: Prentice-Hall.

Peloquin, S. (1990). The patient-therapist relationship in occupational therapy: Understanding visions and images. *American Journal of Occupational therapy, 44,* 13-21.

Rogers, C. (1951). *Client-centered therapy.* Boston: Houghton-Mifflin.

Rogers, C. (1961). *On becoming a person.* Boston: Houghton-Mifflin.

Slagle, E.C. (1922). Training aides for mental patients. *Archives of Occupational Therapy, 1*, 11-17.

Yerxa, E. (1967). Authentic occupational therapy. *American Journal of Occupational Therapy, 21,* 1-9.

Yerxa, E. (1978). The philosophical base of occupational therapy. In American Occupational Therapy Association, *Occupational therapy: 2000 AD*. Rockville, MD: American Occupational Therapy Association.

Yerxa, E. (1991). Seeking a relevant, ethical and realistic way of knowing for occupational therapy. *American Journal of Occupational Therapy, 45,* 199-204.

CHAPTER 2

Establishing Trust

KEY TOPICS	
• Therapeutic relationship	• Psychotropic medications
• Patient rights	• Team relationships
• Paranoia	• Role of occupational therapy in treatment setting
• Differing points of view on patient behavior	

Initial Comments

In our preceding story and discussion, we touched on the issues of a client's right to refuse intervention and the service provider's right to terminate treatment. In that story, the practice setting is the client's residence, and it is fairly easy for the client to refuse intervention. In contrast, in the next story, the patient is in treatment in an inpatient, geropsychiatric setting.

Although the individual described in this story is in treatment voluntarily, she now finds herself in an unfamiliar hospital milieu, and not in the familiar context of her own home. This, plus the new rules she must follow, understandably contribute to her feeling less in charge than she would at home. The occupational therapist in this story does not identify his or her frame of reference but speaks of trying to be "empathetic," and describes a strategy of trying to get into the patient's phenomenological world, suggesting a humanistic orientation. In contrast with the events depicted in the previous story, the therapist seems to feel constrained in his or her ability to carry out a client-centered practice. This may be, in part, because other staff in this setting interpret the client's behavior differently than the occupational therapist does, and perhaps they have different ways of prioritizing their intervention. Contributing to the therapist's anxiety is that he or she is a relative newcomer to the setting, having been employed there for less than a month.

Again the central figure is one who some perceive as "paranoid." If, in fact, this individual is not assessing her situation accurately, then activities would be used to help her with reality testing. Giving her accurate information is vital. Whatever her concerns, it is important that she be cognizant of her choices. Furthermore, she might need someone to advocate on her behalf. As in the previous story of Jane, because the patient is viewed as "paranoid" by staff, there is a tendency by some to dismiss or at least downplay her concerns.

Psychiatric Practice Within a Biomedical Model

This story may make some readers uncomfortable as it discusses the use of medications and restraints. The narrating therapist mentions that most of the patients in this facility have been diagnosed with major depression or are agitated; many have complicating physical problems and are treated with medication that often results in drowsiness. Although we do not know what medications are being administered or why, we read that most of the patients appear highly sedated. It is not unusual for patients in treatment to become distressed when they look around and see others who are medicated or acting in a disturbed fashion. Comments such as "I don't belong here" or "I'm not sick like these other people" sometimes are made. It is often very distressing, too, for family members to see their loved one in a setting where he or she appears to have diminished control or is pleading to go home. Often, concerns are especially high when an individual is first admitted because he or she, as well as the family, may lack information or a context with which to understand what is observed.

As you read this story, we ask you to think about how things might look to you if you were a patient in this setting, and how you would prioritize your actions if you were the therapist in this story. The story we title "Marilyn."

"Marilyn" (Anonymous)

Marilyn was a 70-year-old woman who had never married, had no surviving family members, and had been living alone in an assisted-living retirement community. She was admitted with a diagnosis of major depression to the geropsychiatric unit where I had recently been employed. She had a history of depression, and recently had exhibited decreased interest in activities, reduction in self-care, and increased frequency of tearful episodes. Marilyn also had a large goiter, about the size of an orange, on the side of her neck. She usually wore a turtleneck, making it less obvious to the casual observer. She had stated that she "hated" the way it looked but was afraid of surgery. One of her issues centered around whether to have surgery to remove it.

The unit where Marilyn was a patient was a 20-bed closed psychiatric unit in a general hospital, not locked, but monitored by an electronic security system. The psychiatric unit is run by a national contract corporation which specializes in care for elderly persons who have a primary psychiatric diagnosis, as well as multiple past or current physical/medical problems. The nursing services were provided by the hospital management, program administration and social work by the national elder care corporation, and occupational and physical therapies through contractual service with an outside agency. As the occupational therapist, I was responsible to two contract managers: one a physical therapist and the other a specialist in learning disability who had additional training in elder care and contract management programming. The stated mission of the geropsychiatric unit was to improve the quality of life for seniors through holistic health care and consultation and education to families and members of the senior community.

Most clients were admitted to the program from nursing homes, board and care settings, and retirement communities. Many people, like Marilyn, were referred because of decreased activity, decreased interest in personal self-care, tearfulness, or expressions of a desire to die. Additionally, many came because of agitation and hostile verbal and/or physical behavior toward staff or other residents in the setting in which they had been living. All patients had past or current medical problems such as urinary tract infection, diabetes, chronic obstructive pulmonary disease, high blood pressure, cerebral vascular accident, a history of cardiac arrest, or organic brain syndrome.

The average length of stay for a patient was 4 weeks, during which time staff were to evaluate and adjust the patient's medication regime, evaluate the status of current medical and functional problems and the level of care needed, and monitor the patient's performance in the therapeutic milieu. Patients were expected to be up and dressed for 8 a.m. breakfast in the dining room, to participate in three or more milieu groups, and to remain out of bed and in the dayroom at least 75% of the day (from approximately 8 a.m. to 4 p.m.), Monday through Friday. Most patients participated in physical therapy once or twice a day for mobility and gait training. Milieu groups were led by social workers and occupational therapists. Occupational therapy groups included music, exercise, horticulture, grooming, reminiscence, task, and recreation groups. The groups were run primarily by the occupational therapy assistant. Each patient was evaluated by the occupational therapist who followed the contract occupational therapy protocol, in which the evaluation was based on observation of patient performance during milieu groups and interview with the patient and his or her family. The interview information and observations were recorded on an admission and discharge form. Specific goals usually addressed length of attention to task, level of assistance or independence in self-care tasks, the extent of participation in one or more milieu therapy groups, effective/appropriate expression of personal needs, and initiation of activity. Patient progress was noted weekly in a narrative note in the physician's progress note section of the chart.

I had been employed at this center for less than a month when Marilyn pulled me aside in the hallway to say, "I'm being held against my will...Can you help me get out of here?" Ironically, we were standing right by the front door, a doorway she couldn't step through without setting off an alarm. She went on to say, "My medicine isn't helping me. Look at me, I'm worse. And look at everyone else. They look awful, too." As I looked at her and around the room, I had to agree. Everyone appeared heavily medicated, and most patients couldn't keep their eyes open, even to eat. Many who had walked in willingly were now in wheelchairs with soft restraints to keep them from falling.

I listened to her concerns and tried to empathize with what she seemed to be feeling. I responded by assuring her that staff meant her no harm. I identified for her three options that I felt she had: to discuss her desire for discharge with her physician, to speak to the program director regarding her concerns, or to identify a friend, since she had no family, with whom she could discuss her concerns. Having done this, I tried to refocus her attention on the grooming group for which I was currently responsible, and in which she was scheduled to participate. My response was intended to be supportive and let her know that I understood her concerns, while giving her accurate information about the setting and her options.

She seemed quite passive, so I wasn't surprised when she responded by saying that it would "do no good" to talk to her doctor, because he never spent more than "5 minutes a day" with her. I didn't know whether or not it would do any "good," as she said, but most physicians spent a very brief amount of time daily with their patients. The physician's primary role was monitoring medication dosage. Most patients only could give brief responses to questions or follow one- to two-step instructions. Therefore, physicians usually observed their patients briefly and then sought information from therapists and nurses regarding changes in function.

Marilyn verbalized reluctance to speak to the program director, and basically asked me to do that on her behalf. I went on to my occupational therapy group, in which she had been participating, but on this particular day she did not attend.

Shortly after all this happened, I saw the program director and advised him of the patient's dissatisfaction. He dismissed her concerns with, "Oh, Marilyn—she's paranoid," and proceeded to review for me a description of paranoid delusions, as if I knew nothing about paranoia. My conversation with Marilyn came to the attention of nursing staff, who interpreted her conversation with me as a "bid for one-on-one attention" when she "should have been in group." As far as I know, she never did speak to the program director, nor did he check back with her.

I have been reevaluating my response in this situation. I am not convinced that Marilyn's statements merely reflected paranoia. I had treated her for 3 weeks and had not seen evidence of paranoia before, nor was there a history of paranoid behavior. However, even if she was paranoid, I would respond similarly. The only change is that I would not advise her to see the program director as I felt I had been reprimanded for this. In retrospect, I also needed to find out about the protocol in this setting regarding patient rights. I know there is a statement of patient rights in each patient's chart and a staff person is to review this document with every individual. What I saw on many of these documents, where the patient was to sign his or her name, was a statement to the effect that, "The patient is unable to sign." My current impression is that the rights are also posted on the wall. The question I continue to ask myself is, "Whether or not patients are paranoid, don't they still have the right to be heard, and should similar protocol be followed in any setting, regardless of patient diagnoses and symptoms?"

Discussion Questions

1. What were your thoughts and feelings as you read this story?
2. What practice themes emerge from this story?
3. Put yourself in Marilyn's place and speculate why you might conclude that you or others were being held against your will.
   a. Assuming that Marilyn was not held against her will, what might staff, including the occupational therapist, do to help avoid this kind of misinterpretation?
   b. How would you have responded to Marilyn's concerns?
4. What are the national, state, and facility protocols for patient rights in your community? Where are they published? How do you and a patient or client find out about them?
5. The narrating therapist, administrator, and nursing personnel all seem to perceive Marilyn differently. What are these differences and how might they be accounted for?
6. How does the narrator seem to feel regarding the administrator's response? The nursing staff's response?
7. How would you respond to the administrator or bring about a change of protocol if you believed such a change was warranted?
8. If you were this therapist and you wanted to work comfortably within in the setting in which Marilyn was treated, with the personnel described, what do you believe would need to occur or change?
9. Many of the patients in this setting are medicated and have the responses described. How might the effect of medications impact their occupational therapy treatment as they participate in a grooming group?
10. What are some of the major sedating medications?
    a. To whom are they given and why are they used?
    b. What are their primary side effects?
11. What are some of the major central nervous system stimulants?

a. To whom are they given and why are they used?

b. What are their primary side effects?

12. What criteria would you apply for a patient's participation in an occupational therapy group if you knew he or she was taking medication?
13. What events or statements made in the story of Marilyn point to a client-centered philosophy of practice?

Impressions

BB: When Marilyn says she's being "held against (her) will," she creates an image of being captive or imprisoned—decidedly not an image that connotes a positive therapeutic set toward her treatment. I've long felt there is much wisdom in Maslow's hierarchy. This woman doesn't seem to feel safe and as long as she, in her perception, is being held against her own wishes and perceives others and herself as "getting worse," I wouldn't expect her to pay attention to much else. Further, even though the therapist assures the patient that no one intends her any harm, I'm not convinced by this narrative that the therapist feels comfortable working in this setting. For me, this becomes as much a story about the therapist as it is about the patient. Neither one seems certain that they are in a safe place; I'm speaking of psychological safety as much as physical.

In my estimation, the therapist has several problems to solve. Among these are: "How do I, as part of a treatment team, help the patient to understand the goings-on here, in order that the setting not seem like such a threatening place?" and "What can I do to help her feel that she is not powerless?" then "How can I take care of myself, clarify what I need to know, and articulate my concerns?" In terms of the occupational therapist's interaction with the program administrator, we can identify several areas which may be generating conflict. These could include differences in values, differences in how information is interpreted, and possibly some conflicts around communication and the way roles are understood.

In most biomedical settings like the one described in this narrative, medication plays an important part. All staff must understand and be comfortable with the use of medication, and help clients understand its use. Otherwise, it can be very frightening for clients, as it has been for Marilyn. I wonder if anyone has explained to Marilyn what some of the side effects of her and others' medication might be. Or, if it has been explained, the extent to which she comprehended the information she was given. Sometimes, we give our patients and clients a great deal of information, but in the newness of everything that is going on around them, they really don't understand the information at that time. I know I have had clients and patients tell me that their medication makes them feel "horrible" and I can see that they appear groggy or depressed. I encourage them to speak to their physicians and will often communicate with the physician myself. One of the services we can provide in the comprehensive treatment of our clients is to provide information about the effect that medication is having on daily performance. Marilyn seems to feel very powerless in her current situation and I am concerned, also, about the extent to which she has been involved in determining her own treatment goals and course.

The tension in this story seems created in part by the therapist's working in a setting in which his or her perceptions and actions appear out of sync with those of other staff, and perhaps the philosophy of the unit overall. It's difficult these days to find a treatment setting that functions exclusively within a single frame of reference or model of practice. In hospitals, for instance, staff and referring physicians have experiences drawn from diverse settings and may look at patient problems differently. Situations can arise in which staff members disagree about how best to respond to particular clients or patients. Overall, though, when there's a multidisciplinary team approach, everyone needs to pull in the same direction. By being empathic, hearing out, and perhaps even validating the client's concerns, the narrator pulls in a direction quite opposite from the nursing personnel and the program director. Given the information we have, and understanding that it's from the narrator's perspective, it doesn't seem that other staff are especially client-centered in their responses.

MAB: It seems the staff members described have a biomedical behavior framework. Although the staff would probably say that they are client-centered, I can't get a sense of humanism in the story. In general, I feel that humanism and a client-centered approach are compatible with the frame of reference of the story of Marilyn, as well as with other frames of reference. I tend to use cognitive behavior approaches rather than just behavioral because they easily enhance client-centered goals. After considering a client's ability or functional level, I give explanations at the level of his or her understanding.

The major conflict with the behavioral theories and a client-centered approach may be in staff's interpretations of them. There have been instances where I have been criticized by other staff because, in their view, I was not following the (behavioral) program. However, I openly shared my concerns about the program, and told them what I felt I could realistically implement given my beliefs and view of my responsibility as a therapist. Some staff just looked at me sympathetically as if to say, "You'll understand someday." I have gotten these responses, for instance, on some occasions when I posed alternatives for treatment, from therapists who were suggesting behavior modification programs for clients who presented behaviors that were difficult to manage.

That Marilyn "pulls the therapist aside" to verbalize her concern reminds me that with increased frequency I hear residents of skilled nursing facilities express fear about being seen as someone who complains. They fear that staff will hold it against them and then staff will not attend to their needs. Again this could be "paranoia" or it may be an instance of a staff member wanting to avoid a patient who has been labeled problematic, difficult, or a complainer. Sometimes residents share their concerns or complaints and they seek my assurance that this will be kept in confidence. They say, "I don't want to cause problems." Given that I have not consistently been employed in these settings, I haven't been able to validate or dispute what residents described to me, but I do listen to their concerns.

During the past 5 years, in a variety of settings, I have seen patient rights documents posted in one or more places: near facility entrances, in patients' rooms, in bathrooms, in cafeterias, and near nursing stations, just to name a few. They are in English or in foreign languages, and tend currently to be printed on brightly colored paper to grab attention. Rights brochures also may be given to patients and/or their families. I see them in or on bedside tables.

I recall two recent occasions in which patients were wanting to leave the treatment setting. In the first situation, the charge nurse overheard the resident's desire to leave and my suggestion to this resident that she speak to her physician. Later, the nurse pulled me aside, somewhat angrily, and showed me a sign (visible to staff only) exhibited in the nurses' station which identified the protocol to follow when residents express a desire to leave. The protocol identified the chain of command (nursing director then social worker then program director, etc.) and gave guidelines for calling a family member or advocate.

More recently, when working for a day in a free-standing rehabilitation unit (a step down setting where patients are medically stable and stay an average of 2 weeks maximum), I was evaluating a newly admitted patient who was recuperating from a laminectomy at L3-L4. When I entered the room, she let me know how irritated she was: "I just heard the market dropped yesterday and I can't even find out what's going on in here!" Her first question to me was, "How do I get out of here before I get sick?" She went on to say, "I want to go home. I have neighbors who can look in on me. This isn't a hospital...That man with the mask is infectious and he is out in the hallway..." She then proceeded to describe her medical history with its numerous surgeries, and the vitamin and health routine she followed to stay healthy. She was convinced that she would get sick from being in this setting. As I listened to her concerns and simultaneously evaluated her functional status, I advised her to speak to her physician. Her response was, "How can I do that? This room doesn't even have a phone. If I would have known that, I would have brought my cell phone." I told her that when we were done with her therapy, I would find out the protocol for reaching one of her physicians (surgeon or general practitioner).

When I went to inquire about the location of a phone and her physician's number, staff responses were informative on two accounts: (1) staff had already labeled her as "demanding and difficult" and were glad that I was willing to work with her and (2) there was a portable telephone in the nursing station which I could take to her in her room.

I then reviewed her chart to find her physician's telephone number. The name she gave me was not the one identified on her chart as the person responsible for monitoring her care in this setting. The only note regarding the physician she identified suggested that she would see the patient post-surgery in 3 weeks at her office. Therefore, I returned to this new patient with telephone in hand and advised her of my findings. She was pleased that she could use the phone, but irate that the physicians whom she had known and seen for years were not monitoring her care. Rather, she felt she was under the supervision of a "stranger." Given her dissatisfaction, I dreaded telling her the rest of the news, that the physician monitoring her program visited the center one time per month. Well, I did tell her and her response to me was, "Okay, tell me what I need to do in therapy (occupational and physical) to show you I can get out of here. You are the only one who can help me." I told her I was not permanent staff but the physical therapist was, and that he, as her case manager, could assist her in communication and discharge planning.

We worked for 3 days, in which she demonstrated all the skills needed for a safe discharge to home. As she prepared for discharge, she asked if I did private work and I advised her that the center would refer her to a home care agency. "But are they going to tell me what I have to do and not listen to what I need?" she asked.

CHAPTER 3

Assessing Safety

KEY TOPICS	
• Allen's cognitive disability model	• Kohlman Evaluation of Living Skills
• Cognitive levels	• Discharge planning
• Allen's Cognitive Level test	
• Safety and guardianship	

Initial Comments

We shared the story of Marilyn from our preceding chapter with occupational therapist Martina M. Cooper, OTR/L, who was at that time a graduate student at Colorado State University on a leave of absence to pursue her advanced degree. Tina shared with us her perspective and in the process she described a client with whom she had worked, and who presents a contrast to Marilyn.

The facility where the following took place was also a geropsychiatric inpatient program, and one where many participants had additional physical problems. The intervention framework for occupational therapy at this facility was Claudia Allen's cognitive disability model.

Allen's Cognitive Disability Frame of Reference: Determining Cognitive Level

As you may be aware, occupational therapist Claudia Allen proposes that occupational therapy's predominant role in health care is in the assessment of cognitive function, in particular, cognitive function as it impacts the ability to do everyday tasks and to live independently and safely. Allen's model addresses especially the problems and concerns that arise with those individuals experiencing cognitive disability. Cognitive disability is most often associated with major affective disorders, dementias, schizophrenia, or traumatic brain injury. These disorders are believed to be related to neurological problems that are not expected to improve, except as might occur as a result of a natural healing process or as an outcome of medication. Allen emphasizes that clients who have a cognitive disability cannot be expected to increase their cognitive level once it has stabilized; therefore, participation in occupational therapy will not impact cognitive level (Allen, 1985; Allen, Earhart, & Blue, 1992). In order to more accurately assess a client's cognitive level and the extent of his or her disability, Allen and colleagues (1992) have devised and modified a multi-level scale that ascribes a cognitive level as it relates, in part, to the individual's ability to use cues, attend and engage purposefully over time, imitate others, follow varying kinds of instructions, and plan ahead and anticipate problems. The Allen Cognitive Level test (ACL) is a screening tool that employs this scale to identify a client's cognitive level. Using the ACL, the client is asked to imitate three leather lacing stitches which are demonstrated by the assessor. These are the running (or sewing) stitch, the whip stitch, and the single cordovan. Each stitch is done three times or until the client makes an error that he or she cannot correct. Given the individual's performance on the ACL, a cognitive level is identified. The cognitive levels are scored from a range of 0.9 to 6.0, with a total of 52 potential scores. The lowest scores (Levels 1 to 2) indicate severe disability and need for maximum caregiver assistance; the highest score indicates normal sensorimotor cognitive processing, or the absence of cognitive disability. Scores within the range of Levels 3 through 5 suggest that the individual will need some caregiver assistance in order to live safely within the community. Allen writes that an advantage of the ACL is that it can be used to "quickly assess Levels 3, 4, and 5" (Allen, 1992, p. 10).

Allen and associates have developed other assessment tools, in particular the Routine Task Inventory (RTI) and the Cognitive Performance Test (CPT). The RTI employs a similar multi-level scale to identify cognitive skill level as demonstrated within 20 self-care and instrumental activities of daily living (IADL) tasks (Heimann, Allen, & Yerxa, 1990). The CPT is a newer instrument specifically designed to assess cognitive capacities and limitations in patients with dementia (Levy, 1992). It is composed of six tasks: dressing, shopping, using the telephone, making toast, washing, and traveling. Rather than stopping when the client has difficulty performing a particular skill, the CPT incorporates the systematic addition or exclusion of sensory cues that might influence task performance. In addition to using these assessment instruments, the therapist observes the patient's task performance within the intervention setting, looking for any changes in level of function (Allen, 1985; Allen et al., 1992).

Allen's work (1985) has been strongly influenced by the medical (disease) model. More recently, she has emphasized the incapacitation that is the outcome of disease using the World Health Organization's (1980) system for classifying impairments, disabilities, and handicaps (Allen et al., 1992).

Intervention

Intervention occurs within four phases. The acute phase includes evaluation and treatment of physical sequela, protection from harm, and the evaluation of changes in cognitive level. During the second, or "post-acute" phase, cognitive level will stabilize and optimum cognitive level can be estimated. It is during the post-acute phase of intervention that the therapist can predict the likely level of caregiver support that the individual will need to function safely at discharge (Allen et al., 1992, pp. 20-21).

The third phase of intervention is the rehabilitative phase. At this stage, medical and cognitive improvement have stabilized. Intervention is aimed at improving the client's safety and ability to perform by providing adaptive equipment, making environmental modifications, and teaching caregivers to provide structure and supervision as needed to ensure the client's safety. Toward this goal, an additional role of the occupational therapist may be to advocate within the legal system for the patient or client who is not capable of functioning safely and is unable to manage his or her own affairs (Allen et al., 1992, pp. 22-23). The fourth and final phase is the provision of supportive, ongoing programs (i.e., community activity programs) through long-term care. The persons identified as appropriate for this service have been or are expected to be cognitively disabled for more than 6 months (Allen et al., 1992, p. 16). (The reader may wish to refer to Chapters 8, 9, 12, and 13, in which other cognitive approaches for occupational therapy are illustrated and discussed.)

Gathering Additional Information

The narrator in this story indicates that she has used information from the Kohlman Evaluation of Living Skills (KELS). The KELS is not an assessment instrument identified with Allen's model. Rather, it is an assessment of basic living skills, developed by Linda Kohlman Thomson. Originally developed for an acute, psychiatric setting, it also is used with people with developmental disabilities, adolescents, and often with the elderly. Like the ACL, information from the KELS is used to assist in making a determination about the need for legal guardianship and to help with discharge planning. The KELS tests 17 basic living skills organized under five broad areas: (1) self-care, (2) safety and health, (3) money management, (4) transportation and telephone, and (5) work and leisure. The KELS gathers information through several means, including client self-report (e.g., the client tells what he or she would do in an identified situation), performance of specific living skills within a simulated setting (e.g., the client is asked to make change for a simulated purchase), and observation of the client's appearance. For each skill identified, the client is given a rating of either "Independent" or "Needs Assistance." Recognizing that some items on the assessment are performance based while others are knowledge based, Thomson encourages occupational therapists to supplement information from the KELS with that obtained through other means when making discharge recommendations (McGourty, 1988, p. 140).

The narrative that follows illustrates how the therapist applies Allen's model and brings in data from the KELS to make an important decision. The vignette begins and concludes with the narrator's reflection.

"Ben" Narrated by Martina M. Cooper, OTR/L

I know it's really hard for all of us to deal with issues around patient rights and we are conscious of not restricting someone more than he or she needs to be. I remember one time I worked with a gentleman, "Ben," who had some cognitive dysfunction from a mild, unspecified dementia. He also had physical problems resulting from an earlier hip fracture, and he drank intermittently, which contributed to his dysfunction. We used Allen's model and the ACL to help determine patient ability to function safely at home. Ben wanted to go back home, which for him was an apartment downtown. I tested him using the ACL and he scored at a level of 4.4, which is pretty low to be living home alone. I view the ACL as a screening tool, and given his score I felt that it was important to have him also do the KELS. I like combining information from the ACL and KELS. I think of the ACL as telling about the ability for new learning, while the KELS gives information about old knowledge and the ability to perform specific daily living tasks.

Ben did well on the KELS. His security apartment was subsidized by Housing and Urban Development and had built-in safety features in the bathroom. I talked with him about what living at home entailed. Although it was a bit of a borderline situation, it seemed to me that he would be safe at home as long as he didn't try to cook. That was the one area where I feared his safety could be compromised. So, I took him aside and basically said, "Look, Ben, I think you'll be fine at home as long as you don't do any cooking and aren't drinking. How about you treat yourself, and eat your cooked meals out? You've worked hard and that's something you can do for yourself." I knew that he was financially able to manage this. We talked a bit more and he agreed to this enthusiastically, so I recommended that he go home, not to a more supported living environment. Ben's alcohol and physical problems had been monitored by his geriatrician, who he would continue to see. His family wanted him to live as independently as possible, and they agreed to check on him to make certain he was getting out and eating his meals. I still see him occasionally and he seems to be happy and doing fine, so I'm really pleased.

Sometimes it's pretty clear that patients aren't going to be safe on their own, and family members want to set up some kind of conservatorship or guardianship. In the state I'm from, however, it's a difficult and expensive process that most families don't want to go through. The occupational therapist might be called on to testify about the patient's function, but the patient has to be in extreme danger or really bad off before the court will consider conservatorship. Many times we see patients go home who we know aren't safe, but there's nothing we can do about it.

Discussion Questions

1. In the story of Marilyn from the preceding chapter and in this story, four means of gathering assessment data are identified that are used to make a determination about a client's readiness for discharge and as to the best placement for him or her. Those assessments were: (1) an interview with the client and his or her family, (2) observation of performance in occupational therapy groups and on the living unit, (3) the ACL, and (4) the KELS.
   a. If viewed in isolation, what does each assessment method seem to best capture? What does each miss?
   b. Identify other assessment instruments, methods, or activities used by occupational therapists that you believe are well suited to this goal of evaluating readiness for discharge and making recommendations for placement.
2. How does the therapist narrating this story seem to view the client, Ben? How does this influence her interaction with him?
3. Refer to the story of Marilyn in the preceding chapter. The therapist narrating the story of Marilyn is uncomfortable with the outcome of intervention, while the narrating therapist in the vignette about Ben is comfortable. Identify at least two factors that could account for this disparity.
4. The narrating therapist refers to seeing Ben after his discharge from treatment. What activities and in what context might the therapist have the client perform in order to assess whether or not Ben is safe and functioning well at home?
5. What recommendations would you make to Ben's family that would enable them to help him remain safe in his own home?
6. Assume for a moment that you are in a situation like the one with Ben, and from the ACL scores, you had a "borderline" situation. You need specific examples of performance that you can share with the client's family to support the recommendations that you will make. Cite three specific activities, as examples, that you feel the client should perform safely to demonstrate that he or she is safe at home.

Impressions

BB: The narrator's comments reflect on the fine line between trying to maintain an individual's safety while being the least restrictive. Whether it is in anticipation of presenting our information in the legal system, or more generally, to judge if our clients will be safe in the settings where they will live, it is a priority that occupational therapists establish a firm basis on which to make recommendations for post-treatment placement. I am always concerned that, as therapists, we use what clients and their families tell us. If we're client-centered, that data should be very important. I'm guessing that in the instance of Ben, part of what enabled a successful transition back home was that Ben wanted to return home and his family supported his independence. When families don't support the patient's or client's desire to be independent, things may move very differently.

I have heard and read about many other instances where both the ACL and the KELS were used with a client, as these assessments were viewed as providing complementary information about the client's cognition as well as performance.

Not only are there physical performance and safety issues to consider, but emotional safety concerns as well. We don't want our clients to be humiliated, shamed, or victimized emotionally. I remember, for instance, a woman whom I worked with quite a number of years ago. This woman was a university professor. She was an exceptionally intelligent woman, single, and had a close network of friends. About once a year for many years, her life would be interrupted by a psychotic break. She would become totally incoherent. During these episodes, she would disrobe in public, use profanity, and was somewhat combative. Once recovered, she was soft-spoken, articulate, and very insightful. Over the years, she and her friends had been able to discern some hints in her behavior that preceded a break. When these hints emerged, they would notify her physician and whisk her away to a protective environment—in this instance, a private psychiatric setting. They were concerned that she would do something to embarrass herself and compromise her position at the university. Treatment in large part consisted of waiting for her thinking to clear. Usually that occurred over 10 days, and she then became her former coherent self. This would be an instance of recovery which Allen's model describes well. But she had many esteem issues: she felt badly about herself and was always concerned that someone other than close friends had witnessed her behavior.

MAB: This story is filled with important topics related to the decisions and recommendations that occupational therapists make daily. Evaluating the ability and safe performance of clients requires the skills and expertise of the therapist, sensitivity to family concerns, and a consideration of financial and social supports. The therapist in this story considers all of these issues before making her recommendation for Ben's return home.

I am pleased that the therapist uses more than one assessment to gather data on Ben's performance. The ACL is a quick assessment which meets the limited time allowed for evaluation, given some reimbursement guidelines. However, as the narrator says, it assesses the ability for new learning. Many of the tasks that adults perform at home, a familiar environment, are automatic and do not require new learning. Therefore, an additional evaluation tool is needed. The KELS can give the information to assess the potential for self-care in the home.

Ideally, we would see the patient perform in his or her home environment, but in many settings, third party payers no longer reimburse for home visits. Or, if they do, they reimburse occupational therapy or physical therapy but not both, and usually only for recommending environmental changes in the bathroom. Therefore, therapists may provide literature or draw diagrams, which they leave with families, to describe adaptation recommendations for the home.

Ben is fortunate to have a family who can provide ongoing support for his return home and to have the financial resources available for eating out. When these supports are not available, the therapist might be able to tap into community resources such as Meals on Wheels, or take advantage of home care programs which provide visitation in the home.

My last comments concern the therapist's belief that Ben will not cook. Given that Ben has a cognitive impairment, I am not comfortable with his commitment to "not cook." I don't doubt that he is being honest in his statement, but it is too easy for one's automatic responses to overpower one's good judgment. When in a familiar environment, he may feel safe and assume that he can make a pot of coffee or fix a light meal. Or, when he returns home to his normal routine, he may get out of bed and automatically go to the kitchen and make coffee. Perhaps his stove should be disconnected or small appliances removed—with his and his family's approval, of course.

In general, I find that most patients are desperate to return home and will agree to almost any request from the family, physician, or therapist. Patients often assume that they will need help only temporarily, and many assume that their neighbors, friends, and family will be able to provide that assistance. Therapists need to explore what support is available and assess how realistic these expectations might be.

References

Allen, C.K. (1985). *Occupational therapy for psychiatric diseases: Measurement and management of cognitive disabilities.* Boston: Little, Brown.

Allen, C.K. (1992). Cognitive disabilities. In N. Katz (Ed.), *Cognitive rehabilitation: Models for intervention in occupational therapy.* Boston: Andover.

Allen, C.K., Earhart, C.A., & Blue, T. (1992). *Occupational therapy treatment goals for the physically and cognitively disabled.* Rockville, MD: American Occupational Therapy Association.

Heimann, N.E., Allen, C.K., & Yerxa, E.J. (1990). The routine task inventory: A tool for describing the functional behavior of the cognitively disabled. *Occupational Therapy Practice, 1,* 67-74.

Levy, L. (1992). The use of the cognitive disability frame of reference in rehabilitation of cognitively disabled older adults. In N. Katz (Ed.), *Cognitive rehabilitation: Models for intervention in occupational therapy.* Boston: Andover.

McGourty, L.K. (1988). Kohlman Evaluation of Living Skills (KELS). In B. Hemphill (Ed.), *Mental health assessment in occupational therapy.* Thorofare, NJ: SLACK Inc.

World Health Organization. (1980). *International classification of impairments, disabilities, and handicaps.* Geneva, Switzerland: Author.

CHAPTER 4

Professional Boundaries

KEY TOPICS

- Ego function
- Psychodynamically based occupational therapy
- Dissociative identity disorder
- Using art in therapy
- Responding to suicidal behavior
- Therapist privacy
- Documentation
- Reimbursement for service

Initial Comments

In our next story, the occupational therapist describes her interaction with a young woman whom she calls Sally. Sally was diagnosed with multiple personality disorder, currently referred to in the *DSM-IV* (American Psychiatric Association [APA], 1994) as dissociative identity disorder. This therapist, who talked with us about her story, indicated that she has remembered Sally, not just because of the striking nature of Sally's disorder, but because she, as the therapist, developed an especially good rapport with Sally. The narrator also stated that she witnessed significant improvement in Sally's behavior over the course of treatment, and felt that occupational therapy was an important contributor to this improvement.

Dissociative Identity Disorder

Dissociative identity disorder has more commonly been referred to as multiple personality disorder. It is one of four dissociative disorders identified in the *DSM-IV* (APA, 1994). As discussed in *Kaplan and Sadock's Synopsis of Psychiatry* (7th ed.) (Kaplan, Sadock,

& Grebb, 1994), the concept of personality suggests integration in the way a person "thinks, feels, and behaves" and an "appreciation of himself or herself as a unitary being" (Kaplan et al., 1994, p. 644). People with this disorder have two or more personalities (referred to as "alters"), each of which organizes attitudes and behaviors during the time period in which it dominates. There is frequently one personality that tends to be the dominant one (sometimes referred to clinically as the "host"), who is identified with the person's legal name. However, there may be no such dominant host. Often, each personality presents a picture quite different, even opposite from the other(s). For example, one personality may be very reserved, another outgoing, or one may be sexually inhibited, a second sexually promiscuous (Kaplan et al., 1994, p. 646). This disorder includes an amnesiac component, with one or more of the personalities unable to remember events that took place while an alter was dominant.

Consistent in the histories of those who have dissociative identity disorder are a traumatic event in childhood, contributing environmental factors, and an absence of external support. The traumatic event is most often physical and/or sexual abuse, frequently incestuous, during childhood. Other contributing events may include the death of a close relative or friend during childhood or witnessing a death or trauma in childhood (Kaplan et al., 1994, p. 644). The environmental factors that impact the development of this disorder are likely to include the lack of positive role models and an absence of available means to obtain support or deal with stress. In other words, the disorder results from the combination of dealing with tremendously stressful circumstances and lacking means to cope. According to statistics, this disorder is most common in late adolescence or young adulthood, with a mean age of diagnosis of 30 years, although individuals with this disorder usually have had symptoms for many years before being diagnosed. People who receive this diagnosis are overwhelmingly women, but researchers speculate that it may be underrecognized in men, who are more likely to enter the criminal justice system than the mental health system. Dissociative identity disorder can develop in very young children, in which case the symptoms may include hallucinatory voices, signs of depression, and self-injurious behavior. Suicide attempts in all age groups are common in persons having this disorder (Kaplan et al., 1994, pp. 644-645).

Intervention with Dissociative Identity Disorder

In this, the decade of the brain, emphasis is being placed on the increased understanding of neurological factors as they influence thinking, feeling, and behaving. Psychotherapy has taken a back seat. Within psychiatry, however, the belief is maintained that the coupling of psychotherapy with neurologic intervention (e.g., medication) often enables the most progress in treatment (Kaplan et al., 1994, pp. vii-ix). In the case of dissociative identity disorder, drug-assisted interview has been used in treatment, but medication is not the primary intervention strategy (Kaplan et al., pp. 646, 648).

A review of the literature indicates that insight-oriented psychotherapy, or what Kaplan and colleagues (1994) refer to as "expressive-supportive psychodynamic therapy," is most effective with this disorder (p. 644). This refers to therapy that pays particular attention to understanding how the individual's personality and coping styles developed. Enhancing insight while helping to support healthier coping are primary goals within this model.

In the following story, the treatment milieu was created by an inpatient, psychiatric, university-affiliated hospital with a strongly psychodynamic orientation. The patients in this setting are of all ages. The length of stay identified for the central figure, Sally, is over 3 months, a time span that might well be viewed as a luxury in our current health care system. What this lengthy hospitalization allows is more intensive psychotherapy. The occupational therapist's intervention strategies include building the client's insight and self-awareness and helping her to identify and appropriately express uncomfortable thoughts and feelings that have been unmanageable for her. The therapist also helps the client build feelings of mastery and coping skills related to everyday tasks. In order to help you orient to this story, we briefly review principles of a psychodynamically based occupational therapy practice with particular reference to dissociative identity disorder.

Nature of the Person in Psychodynamic Theory

In 1963, occupational therapist Gail Fidler and her husband, psychiatrist Jay Fidler, collaborated to write *Occupational Therapy: A Communication Process in Psychiatry*. Several years later, Anne Mosey (1970) followed with her occupational therapy text, *Three Frames of Reference for Mental Health*. These books articulated a psychodynamically based, or what Mosey called an "object relation analysis," framework for occupational therapy practice. It was a practice model closely allied to the psychodynamically based model prevalent in psychiatry at that time. Linking Freudian, Jungian, and neo-Freudian theory to core occupational therapy principles, as articulated by Fidler and Fidler and Mosey, people can be viewed as dynamic energy systems composed of parts known to the self and parts of which one is unaware. In the language of this model, the basis for occupation is the person's participation with human and nonhuman objects, or their object relationships. It is through object relationships that people meet their needs. Tension is created when needs cannot be met; this and the perceived drive toward greater experience are identified as motivators for human behavior, or occupation.

Conceptualizing the Personality

Many metaphorical concepts, including those of "id," "ego," and "superego" and "conscious," "unconscious," and "defenses," have been employed to explain how thoughts and feelings of which people are unaware and events in the past play a significant role in influencing their thoughts, feelings, and occupational style in the present. Freud and early followers emphasized the importance of primitive unconscious motives in determining behavior and of psychosexual developmental stages in determining object choice. More recent literature has emphasized the role of the ego in conscious behavior (Fine, 1979) and in enabling sound function. The ego in particular is responsible for distinguishing real from not real (often referred to as reality testing), making judgments, acting upon feelings in a reasonable way, and governing behavior designed to meet needs. The ego maintains a sense of the self as an integrated whole, and enables the person to be an effective occupational being.

Not everything the ego does is done consciously. Much of the work of the ego is to keep thoughts or feelings repressed, or out of conscious awareness—in particular, thoughts that would make the person anxious. The many defense mechanisms referred to in popular language represent means by which uncomfortable thoughts or feelings can be kept from conscious awareness. In the case of dissociative identity disorder, the ego is overwhelmed by traumatic events and responds by splitting off or, in a sense, disowning unacceptable thoughts, feelings, and behaviors, and giving them to the other personality(s). While this disowning of feelings and behaviors is striking in dissociative disorder, a similar process is suggested in many of the patients and clients treated in occupational therapy. We may see adolescents, for example, who present as angry and belligerent and are relatively out of touch with feelings of sadness and loss regarding their own life experiences. When they can identify that sadness, these young people may become better equipped to ask for what they need from significant people in their lives and control their own behavior.

When individuals are unable to think and behave coherently due to gross impairments in reality testing, and are severely impaired in their ability for occupational performance, the term "psychotic" is commonly applied (Kaplan et al., 1994, p. 325). Psychosis identifies a breakdown in the ability of the ego to function.

Motivation

While traditional psychodynamic theory viewed tension reduction and personal gratification as primary motivators in human activity, the understanding of this broadened and changed in emphasis with the work of such ego psychologists as Robert White (1959, 1971) and Heinz Hartmann (1958). Ego psychology emphasizes that the ego doesn't just serve the id to reduce conflict, but functions autonomously to enable adaptation and mastery within the environment (Hartmann, 1958).

White's work comes to our particular attention in the *American Journal of Occupational Therapy* (1971). White describes the person as possessing an "effectance motivation," or an inner striving to explore and master challenges in his or her world. Once a task is mastered, the person is believed to be compelled to create new challenges, which in turn he or she will strive to master. This is reminiscent of the actualization motive identified by existential humanists.

Health

Healthy or adaptive occupational function includes being able to engage in meaningful occupation in a manner that respects the rights and needs of others and with a relative lack of conflict or anxiety. As indicated, this is primarily directed by the ego. It includes having a positive self-concept, having an accurate assessment of reality, having a repertoire of social and occupational skills, and balancing a concern for others with meeting one's own needs.

Therapeutic Relationship

In the therapeutic relationship in occupational therapy, the therapist collaborates with the patient or client to foster healthy ego functioning. It is believed that in some instances the client will try to recreate in the therapeutic relationship patterns of relating or conflicts that have arisen in previous relationships. In everyday practice, occupational therapists who do not directly identify their practice as psychodynamic often use psychodynamic principles to understand and respond to behavior.

Therapeutic Activity and Environment

Occupation can be the catalyst in facilitating interaction between the patient and others, serve as a vehicle for enhanced self-understanding, provide a reality-based structure, or can be the avenue for skill acquisition or enhancement. Fundamentally, all of these uses of activity support the individual's efforts to be meaningfully engaged in the occupations of his or her life.

The manner in which people carry out tasks and interact while participating in occupational therapy is believed to be very similar to their style of engagement in their non-treatment environment. Participation in occupation, therefore, provides a means for clients and patients to learn (at their level of understanding) about how they approach tasks, to test their own abilities and limits, and to change their way of approaching tasks, if they so choose. Often one's engagement in therapeutic tasks evokes strong feelings. If these are identified and dealt with, people can reach goals more easily.

Speaking again in the language of this model, the less effective a person's ego function, the more the occupational therapist will have to supply ego (i.e., structure the therapeutic environment and the activity, set limits, and assist in decision making). For clients who are internally disorganized or psychotic, activities will be selected that give information at the level the individual can comprehend, and have performance demands consonant with the functioning level of the compromised client.

One of the emphases in the application of a psychodynamic framework is in the area of self-esteem. Many individuals who seek help within the mental health arena have problems related to esteem. Meaningful tasks are used whereby individuals can experience success and begin the process of building a feeling of efficacy and self-worth. This often includes the person seeing himself or herself as an effective problem solver. Occupational therapists therefore often use therapeutic activities to help clients improve in their problem solving (an ego function), as well as using tasks to assess problem solving as clients prepare to terminate therapy or leave the intervention setting.

Kaplan and Sadock's Synopsis of Psychiatry (7th ed.) (Kaplan et al., 1994) identifies a number of basic principles and goals for intervention with dissociative identity disorder. There are several that seem particularly relevant to occupational therapy. As summarized, these are: (1) creating an atmosphere of safety, (2) if the individual engages in destructive or self-destructive behavior, engaging him or her and appropriate personalities in a contract regarding these behaviors, (3) since the condition results from the person feeling overwhelmed, focusing on mastery and the person's active participation in the intervention process, (4) pacing treatment so the individual can integrate new insights difficult to understand and tolerate, (5) addressing and trying to correct cognitive errors on an ongoing basis, (6) helping the person learn new coping skills as the personality merges into a unified whole, and (7) helping the person to "live in the world" (p. 647).

"Sally" Narrated by Mary E. Conrad, MBA, OTR/L

Sally was adopted as a young child, along with one brother. The couple who adopted these siblings lived in the country and the family had numerous animals, mostly dogs and cats. As Sally remembered it, the animals were more important than the children. One of Sally's jobs as a child was to take care of these animals—feeding them, grooming them, and cleaning up after them. Sally said she "loved" the animals, but if she didn't do the job "perfectly," as she described, then she would be hollered at or struck by either parent. Both she and her brother were physically abused throughout their childhood.

Sally was 20 years old when she was brought into the inpatient psychiatric hospital. She had been found hiding behind a bush, covered in blood. Apparently, she had violently killed an animal. As it was learned, Sally had two personalities. The "Sally" personality was docile, did whatever she was told, and was very nuturing. The second personality, whom I'll call "Tracy," would become angry, disappear for brief periods, and kill animals.

When Sally came to occupational therapy, she sometimes came as Sally, sometimes as Tracy. Initially, neither personality seemed to be aware of the other. My goal in occupational therapy was to help her understand and accept her angry feelings, and not have to disown them. Sally liked to draw and do crafts, so I used these as a means for her to express her feelings. Some of her drawings were very decorative, while some were tumultuous-looking with lots of red and black. They usually were designs and patterns, not depictions of events. She seldom had much to say about them, but would take them back to her room. I never suggested anything she should do with them. Because Sally liked to do crafts, I also encouraged her to select craft projects that she enjoyed. It was an area in which she excelled, and she eventually was able to teach some of the other patients who were less skilled. This helped Sally see herself as skilled and having something to offer others. Since I saw my patients in groups and we sometimes did group activities, there were also everyday-type interactions where Sally might have needs she would have to verbalize if they were to be met, or instances in which she would get annoyed or distressed. I could use these as opportunities to help her accept that it's okay to ask for what you need, or to get angry and let people know how you feel. Sally was suicidal when she first came in for treatment, and when she got upset, our suicide precautions with Sally/Tracy increased.

Sally/Tracy was in treatment for several months and gradually began, as Sally, to accept the negative side of herself and to understand that her anger was primarily toward her abusive parents. She also became better able to verbalize her needs and feelings to patients and staff. We began to see less and less of Tracy.

As Sally prepared for discharge, I worked with the social worker to help prepare Sally to gain employment. Throughout this last phase of treatment, Sally was involved in the decision-making process as we worked to identify a place she would like to live and looked toward prospective employment. Following some vocational counseling, it was arranged that she would be trained to do data entry, and would move from the inpatient setting to an adult group residence. One of my final treatment activities with Sally was to go shopping with her and the social worker to help her select a new work wardrobe. Although I had never given Sally my home phone number, we had talked frequently during her hospitalization, and she knew my name and the part of town where I lived.

Sally had been discharged for about a week when I got a call at home. It was about 2:00 a.m., and the call was made by one of the resident staff persons at the halfway house where Sally now lived. Sally had climbed onto the roof of the three-story residence, threatening to jump. This staff person was afraid to call the police, concerned that if Sally saw police, she might get frightened and jump. Sally had asked them to call me, and indicated that she would jump if I didn't come to where she was. She said that she felt scared and unsure of her new life. I responded that I would like to see her in the morning instead. I told her that I knew it was scary, but that she had worked hard in therapy and had the skills she needed. She agreed to come down from the roof, which she did, and to meet me at 9:00 a.m. later that morning. The resident manager where she lived said he would check on her during the night, and that he would notify her psychiatrist of what had occurred.

I didn't sleep very well that night. The fact is, I would have come over if she had not agreed to come off the roof and meet me later that day.

Sally showed up for our 9:00 a.m. meeting, tearful but otherwise all right. She again talked about feeling frightened of being on her own, but left affirming that she was going to give it a try. I heard over the next several months that she was employed and doing well.

Discussion Questions

1. The occupational therapist narrating this story indicates that the use of crafts and drawing provided a vehicle for this client to express feelings. Identify two occupational therapy theoretical assumptions upon which the therapist based her decision to use expressive activities.

2. Describe specific activities/media or ways that multiple media could be used which would facilitate the expression of feelings and how they would be used.
3. Identify how you would communicate this as part of a functional (performance) outcome in writing your treatment goals.
4. Identify cautions or concerns you as the therapist would have if using expressive activities with an individual like Sally/Tracy.
5. The narrating therapist also indicates that she used Sally's interest in crafts plus "everyday-type" group activities to give Sally an arena for building confidence and asking for what she needed. Describe how you might use group tasks to facilitate this kind of learning for Sally.
6. What could you, as the occupational therapist, do to help create a safe and supportive environment in which needs, thoughts, feelings, and concerns could be expressed and integrated by an individual such as Sally?
7. The narrator writes that at times during her hospitalization, suicide concerns increased for Sally. What precautions might you take when working with an individual who is believed to be at risk for suicide?
8. In the intervention settings with which you are familiar, how are staff members identified (e.g., first name only, first and last name, title)?
   a. How does this method of identification reflect the way staff members relate to clients? Is the communication between staff and clients very casual? More formal?
   b. In these settings, is it relatively easy or difficult for clients/patients to contact staff at home?
   c. What are your feelings about having clients/patients know your full name? Calling you at home? Would this depend on the setting in which you were employed?
9. Have you ever been in a situation where an individual having suicidal feelings has contacted you? Describe the situation, including your response and your concerns.
10. Are you comfortable with the decision made by the occupational therapist in response to Sally's phone call? Might you have done something different? If so, what, and based on what reasoning?

Impressions

BB: I'm glad that we have been able to include this story because it illustrates how psychodynamic understanding can contribute to occupational therapy's intervention with psychological disorders. I wonder sometimes if the increased medicalization of mental health care leads people to believe that all psychological problems and problems of living will be solved with the use of medication.

I have a holistic bias that rejects this idea, but I can understand its attractiveness. It seems endogenous to occupational therapy that we view problems of living as calling for more than a medical cure. I have an additional bias which is that it can be very helpful for us as occupational therapists to have a conceptual framework for understanding the hows and whys of human behavior. Several disorders, in particular those associated with trauma, seem well described by the psychodynamic model: dissociative disorder and post-traumatic stress disorder, reactions to abuse in adults and children, and borderline personality disorder. Whatever the disorder and whatever the words we use to describe it, the psychological self is always there.

When I read this story, it seems evident that the therapeutic relationship, use of occupation, and therapeutic milieu all contribute to Sally's improvement, though we have a somewhat sketchy portrait of how this transpired. I want to emphasize that occupational therapy at this setting does not occur in isolation nor does it represent the whole of treatment. The very fact that Sally is in a safe environment, where appropriate boundaries are in place and where she can trust that she won't be allowed to hurt herself or others, enables her to begin managing her feelings, behaviors, and life. Within this context, staff can show her how to ask for what she needs and encourage her efforts at coping. She has something she never had at home—a support system. The narrating therapist recounts the story's most important event—Sally's climb to the rooftop and subsequent call to the occupational therapist. The therapist has to make a decision about how to respond to Sally's telephone call. We don't know everything that the narrator might have weighed as she made that decision, but it undoubtedly included trying to assess Sally's coping skills, the manner in which Sally's safety needs were addressed by the staff with her, and something about the relationship between herself and Sally—and how that would impact Sally's ability to honor an agreement.

I brought this story to my class and they expressed several concerns. One centered around the fact that this therapist and not the psychiatrist was being called by the client. Given that this client has a rapport with the narrator, we can understand how this might happen, even if it doesn't follow the hierarchy of authority that we might expect in treatment. This led to a second concern from the students about being called at home by patients or clients. Their worry was that a potentially dangerous or unstable individual would try to contact them or follow them home. They wondered about their own right to privacy and how that could best be ensured.

Another area that they expressed concern about was whether or not we as occupational therapists could be reimbursed for services where expressing and accepting feelings was a goal. It seems vital that in the initial assessment of Sally, the occupational therapist identify that Sally's difficulty with acknowledging feelings was impeding the integration of the person as a cohesive, functional whole. Then the occupational therapist could make the link between a goal of appropriate expression (and acceptance) of thoughts and feelings, especially anger, to improved function. We read that the expression of negative thoughts and feelings was not the entire occupational therapy goal. Helping Sally learn to ask for what she needed in the course of daily experiences and increasing her sense of mastery were equally important in treatment. These represent something of a package, the longer term goal of which would be Sally's improved occupational function, which the story suggests was achieved.

Students frequently say that they aren't sure what to do when they know what a patient or client needs to achieve, but don't know if the goal is reasonable because it might not be reimbursable. (I suspect that's not only a student concern either.) My response is undoubtedly simplistic, but in principle it's this: you do what the client really needs, then you find a way to document it that will satisfy third party payers. I believe that a sensible fit usually exists between what the client wants for himself or herself, what you as the therapist perceive the client to "need," and what can be justified. Often it's a matter of being very clear ourselves about those connections so we can articulate them well.

Several students also indicated that they wouldn't know what to do if a patient produced artwork that they would have to "analyze." I tried to clarify what they meant by analyze, since I didn't see any analyzing going on in this story. In fact, I was left wondering whether or not the therapist and Sally did talk about her drawings. The class and I were able to talk about the way expressive arts in occupational therapy could or should be used. I suspect that the preparation around this varies among occupational therapy professional curricula and I trust many different philosophies are represented.

MAB: Before responding to documentation and reimbursement issues, I wanted to comment on the students' concern about "analyzing" patient artwork. First of all, I don't analyze art. To me, this means interpreting for the patient what the art means. However, I feel the meaning of the work comes from the artist/patient. Therefore, I would use open-ended questions to elicit the patient's view and increase his or her self-understanding, and help the patient interpret his or her own work and its significance in the "here and now." I am aware of multiple theories for the interpretation of art in therapy, but I do not use these theories to formulate questions. Rather, I use the product as a stimulus for interaction. My initial questions solicit the patient's opinion, such as "Tell me about your drawing" or "What did you learn from the art experience?" or "When you look at your work, what do you feel?" Usually these discussions help the patient achieve insight they can use to cope with current concerns. Within the context of these discussions, I can give the patient feedback in which I may affirm a patient's beliefs or give an alternative view of his or her performance. For instance, when a patient or client is critical of what he or she has produced, I might ask about his or her enjoyment of the process of working with the art medium. Sometimes at the end of the therapy session, I summarize what I have learned about patients within the context of the art experience, and ask them to share their view of the experience. I also use this explorative-feedback approach around other objects produced in occupational therapy. I feel that when art and other objects are created within occupational therapy they become tools for interaction, and the purpose of using activities in therapy is to help patients learn from their experiences. Sometimes patients do not have a clear understanding of the value of tasks used in therapy, or even when they understand the goal of a treatment session, they may not understand how the goal is achieved through a particular task. On more than one occasion I have heard patients refuse cognitive games or tasks, and insist that they need "exercise." Or they comment "Wouldn't my grandchild love to see me do this?" or inquire "Why should I cook?...I can hire someone to help me." Therefore, giving them feedback at the end of the therapy hour can help them link the therapeutic goal and use of the therapeutic task. Feedback of this kind also can act as the basis for writing weekly summaries which identify patient progress. During this therapist/patient exchange, patients can be informed of their progress from the therapist perspective, express their views about their own progress and any concerns, and participate in setting new goals.

As for documentation, I agree that you do what the client really needs, and then find a way to document it. I also agree that reimbursement concerns are not unique to students nor to occupational therapy. I recently have become acquainted with several different documentation guides, one from the AOTA (1995), and I have participated in several documentation inservices. In these sessions, clinicians and administrators have been identifying the fit between patient/client needs, the services provided, and the documentation guides of third party payers. Although there has been some variation in the payers' specific expectations for therapy and documentation for reimbursement, there seems to be an overall fit between client needs and reimbursable service.

References

American Occupational Therapy Association. (1995). Elements of clinical documentation (Rev. ed.). *American Journal of Occupational Therapy, 49,* 1032-1035.

American Psychiatric Association. (1994). *Diagnostic and statistical manual of mental disorders* (4th ed.). Washington, DC: Author.

Fidler, G., & Fidler, J. (1963). *Occupational therapy: A communication process in psychiatry.* New York: Macmillan.

Fine, R. (1979). *A history of psychiatry.* New York: Columbia University Press.

Hartmann, H. (1958). *Ego psychology and the problem of adaptation* (D. Rapaport, Trans.). New York: International Universities Press.

Kaplan, H., Sadock, B., & Grebb, J. (1994). *Kaplan and Sadock's synopsis of psychiatry* (7th ed.). Baltimore: Williams and Wilkins.

Mosey, A.C. (1970). *Three frames of reference for mental health.* Thorofare, NJ: SLACK Inc.

White, R.W. (1959). Motivation reconsidered: The concept of competence. *Psychological Review, 66,* 297-333.

White, R.W. (1971). The urge toward competence. *American Journal of Occupational Therapy, 25,* 271-274.

CHAPTER 5

Confused Behavior

KEY TOPICS

- Kaplan's directive group
- Psychosis
- Reality testing
- Delusional system
- Safety concerns
- Helping client group respond to confused behavior

Initial Comments

In our next story and in the dialogue that follows we address principles for responding to confused or disoriented behavior. What follows is an instance in which the occupational therapist helps a patient with reality testing. The encounter described could have occurred almost anywhere in the treatment facility. Since it occurred during an occupational therapy activity group, we have the opportunity to discuss the potential impact such an encounter has on the occupational therapist's and patient group's feelings of safety and well-being.

The setting for the following narrative is an inpatient, acute care psychiatric setting, with a very brief average length of stay. The narrator writes that occupational therapy occurred in three tiered groups, based on the group model used by Kathy Kaplan, as described in her book *Directive Group Therapy* (1988). Kaplan in turn credits the Model of Human Occupation ([MOHO] Kielhofner, 1985, 1992) as providing a basis for her conceptualization of group organization.

Model of Human Occupation Constructs Used for Tiering Groups

According to Kaplan, and as based on MOHO (Kielhofner, 1985, 1992), patients and clients can be viewed as open systems who take in information from the environment, process it (or think about and integrate the information), and then respond through their performance or behavior (Kaplan, 1988). These individuals vary in their ability to use information and to interact appropriately within the environment. Individuals who are cognitively disorganized, for instance, may have difficulty making sense of the data they take in, and subsequently, they may be unable to generate an appropriate and organized behavior or response. (Although applying MOHO does not require the use of psychodynamic vocabulary, one could draw a parallel here to the discussion of the function of the ego, as described in Chapter 4.) Verbal psychotherapy groups often require participants to have a long attention span and to process abstract verbal dialogue, and therefore are not an appropriate match for the individual who is agitated or confused. Accordingly, occupational therapy treatment groups can be made to match the clients' cognitive and performance abilities. In this model, too, the principle applies that the more disorganized the patients' cognitive processing and behaviors, the more the therapist will need to provide structure and support within the milieu, and the less will be the performance demands of the activities used.

Given this basis, Kaplan identifies three treatment group levels for occupational therapy. These three group levels correspond with the three stages of occupational function identified within MOHO: exploration, competence, and achievement (Kielhofner, 1985). Groups identified as "exploratory" represent the simplest level of challenge and highest degree of external structure, and are aimed at helping patients who are disorganized to learn basic skills. The "directive group" is an example of an exploratory group. The next level of groups, which Kaplan refers to as "competence level groups," are available to individuals who have more internal structure and therefore can collaborate with the therapist in various tasks and activities. What Kaplan calls "achievement level groups" represent the group activity level having the highest performance demand, in which participants will be given the most autonomy (1988, pp. 21-22).

The directive group, as conceived by Kaplan, responds to the needs of the lower functioning client by paying special attention to the level of arousal, degree of interpersonal interaction, level of structure, and other kinds of input and demands made by the group and activities. The purpose of the directive group is to "assist patients in reorganizing their behavior to a basic level of competence" and to thereby prepare "extremely disturbed patients in a short-term setting...(to eventually move on to)...group psychotherapy and activity-oriented groups" (Kaplan, 1988, pp. 22-23).

Therapeutic Response in Psychosis

The severely disturbed or disorganized people to whom the directive group is aimed often show evidence of thought disorder or psychosis. Psychosis traditionally has been defined as an inability to distinguish real from nonreal or fantasy, or the inability to engage in reality testing, which includes understanding information and using it to make sound judgments (Kaplan, Sadock, & Grebb, 1994, p. 304). The person who is psychotic may have disturbances in the content of his or her thoughts. For instance, he or she may have paranoid fears, delusions, or other illogical thoughts not realistically based. Or he or she may have a disturbance in the form of thought which manifests as an inability to organize thoughts and bring them together to problem solve. This is illustrated, for example, by tangential thinking and loose associations, confusion about how to carry out everyday tasks, and inappropriate social and task behavior (Kaplan et al., 1994, pp. 304-305). The inability of psychotic persons to function in daily life presents the challenge to occupational therapists.

When individuals are unable to engage effectively in reality testing, it becomes a role of the therapist or care provider to help them with this process; for instance, by pointing out to the disturbed person that his or her thoughts or conclusions (when verbalized) are not realistic. For example, the therapist may begin his or her comments with a phrase such as, "I realize that this (situation) may not appear so to you, but from my perspective what's going on here is..." This does not mean that every inaccurate observation made by a client must be confronted. The goal in helping the person to engage in reality testing is to provide information in a way that can be managed by the confused individual.

When working with cognitively impaired persons, such as those with dementia, an approach referred to as reality orientation is sometimes used. Reality orientation is an ongoing process closely related to reality testing. When using a reality-oriented approach, therapists consistently remind disoriented persons of names, the day and time, places, and events. To help establish orientation, clocks and calendars may be conspicuously placed. The occupational therapist speaks slowly and clearly, and may supplement speech with nonambiguous nonverbal messages. For example, the therapist might approach a confused Mr. Jones and say, "Hi, Mr. Jones! It's 9:00 and time for the group to go on our walk. It's cold and you will need your sweater," and then hand the sweater to Mr. Jones.

When disturbances in interpreting reality are severe, the client may, understandably, become very frightened. In those instances, the primary goal is to keep the individual safe.

The following story describes an instance where the occupational therapist has helped the client engage in reality testing. We ask you to pay particular attention to how the occupational therapist achieved this, including the therapist's calm manner. This also is a story about the feelings and discomfort of the narrating therapist as she recognizes that she is part of a disoriented person's delusional system. One way we as therapists can cope with difficult situations and uncomfortable feelings is to step back and remind ourselves of our own boundaries. Other people's sadness is not our sadness; their confusion is not our confusion, even though we have empathy for their feelings and problems. After she contributed this story, the narrating therapist told us that it was "chilling" for her when she realized that this patient did not perceive her as separate. This story, unnamed by our contributor, we entitle "Kathy."

"Kathy" Narrated by Martina M. Cooper, OTR/L

The setting for this clinical story is a 13-bed inpatient psychiatric crisis unit. Many of the patients were placed on a doctor's court hold because they were judged to be a threat to themselves, others, or property. The average length of stay was 5 days. One afternoon, I had started the occupational therapy activity group with a small number of people—four patients in total. We were seated around one table in the milieu (or dayroom). Theoretically, all the patients on the unit were eligible for the group as long as they could concentrate on some type of task long enough to participate and be around other people for approximately 45 minutes. This group was modeled after Kaplan's directive group.

The group had started with a warm-up in which members were asked to introduce themselves and recall one activity they like to do in the springtime. After this introductory stage, we discussed the goals of the group and began working on a group collage made up of pictures and words that reflected activities that were relaxing to individual patients. After receiving directions and supplies, the group members worked quietly and intently on the project.

I was in the midst of asking someone about the picture he was cutting out when I heard someone behind me call me "Kathy." I turned around and stated, "My name is Tina and we are in the process of doing an occupational therapy group." The person responded, "Kathy, why are you here? I read in the obituary that you are dead. Why are you doing this to me?" I saw before me a woman in her late 40s or early 50s, dressed in a hospital gown, with a brown beehive hairstyle, staring at me with a blunted affect. She was holding a cup with coffee and slowly walking closer to me. I again repeated my name, and identified the hospital's name and my role, but this time in a much quieter voice. I slowly backed away, glancing toward another occupational therapist working on her notes in a nearby office with a window. I again repeated my name quietly and gently. I began to remember this patient's story—that her name was Kathy, and that she had been found wandering the streets with "voices" telling her to kill herself. Within a few seconds, I felt very frightened. Just as I thought I might walk quickly to the occupational therapy office, Kathy turned and walked away.

Kathy returned to her room. I excused myself from the group and asked my occupational therapy colleague in the office to check with this woman's nurse. Her nurse and the other staff needed to know about the psychotic behavior she was demonstrating and probably needed to reconsider allowing this patient to be out on the ward unsupervised.

When I returned to the group in progress, I was surprised by how little the patients claimed to have noticed. One person said they thought Kathy seemed "confused," but appeared to be assuaged by the fact that Kathy's nurse had been contacted. We finished the collage, and had a simple discussion about the importance of recreation and relaxation.

After the group, I went back to the office and acknowledged more freely to myself how this episode had affected me. I was struck by fear and the eeriness of being in this woman's delusional system. I felt unsafe as I entered her world and tried to imagine how terrifying it must be for her to have no way to test reality, or even to know reality when she was actively psychotic. Initially, I questioned my response to her. I wondered if I should have gone to the office sooner. Upon reflection, I think I used intuition to lead my actions. I had responded slowly because I thought a quicker, louder response would have sent her coffee cup and its hot contents flying at me. I knew she was out in the dayroom, but I didn't know how unstable her ego boundaries were. Generally, the nurses on this ward did an excellent job of titrating patients out of their security room, but this illustrated that no system is perfect.

Discussion Questions

1. The narrating therapist describes feeling fearful and struck by the "eeriness" of her encounter with Kathy. Try to imagine that you were the therapist in this story. How do you think you would have felt?
2. What might you do if you needed some support following this incident?
3. What was there about the setting (physical space as well as procedures) that helped the therapist feel reasonably safe?
4. How do you think this therapist's manner (i.e., her tone of voice) contributed to the outcome of this story?
5. Describe, if you can, a situation where you think your manner did or didn't enhance your ability to keep a situation calm and safe.
6. The other patients in this story seemed not to have been disturbed by the incident they witnessed. Offer some plausible explanation for their lack of concern.
7. Patients may need help to manage the confused behavior of other patients. Staff modeling is one approach for educating patients. Describe and discuss other methods of teaching patients to manage confused or inappropriate behavior exhibited by their peers.

Impressions

MAB: While Kathy's disorientation in this story probably reflects schizophrenia or a delusional disorder, I'm reminded of similar situations where clients have been confused due to dementia or head injury. Some people avoid the confused person, but others can become angry at this individual who may insult them personally or make them feel "crazy," or they may interpret the patient's inappropriate gestures or comments as threatening and become very frightened. Recently I was sitting in a dayroom with six patients and speaking to a 79-year-old woman, Mrs. L., who was hospitalized for depression. She was verbalizing her concerns about an anticipated surgery. She was afraid and critical of herself for being fearful. During the discussion we were distracted by an older gentleman who got up from the sofa and began to wander toward us, mumbling a few incoherent sentences to us. I asked the gentleman to return to his seat and advised him that I or another therapist would be with him in a few minutes. I handed him a colorful *National Geographic* to review as he waited and I returned to the other patient.

When I returned, Mrs. L. said to me, "I don't know how to respond to this man. He doesn't make any sense when he talks, and I can't understand him." Frequently, his speech was incoherent. She then recalled incidents with her spouse (now deceased) who would become angry because she couldn't understand him and couldn't respond to his incoherent requests. She proceeded to describe the strategy she used to communicate with her spouse. She said, "I learned to ask questions that could be answered with 'yes' or 'no'." I suggested that this might be an effective strategy with this gentleman and that we wouldn't know for sure until we tried.

On this same unit, on another occasion, I recall being surprised to see Nina, a small, frail, elderly woman, standing in the dayroom nose to nose with one of our more confused patients, Ella. Nina, who usually was withdrawn and nonverbal, began to holler at Ella, "...if you do that again I'll flatten you..." I'm not sure what the provocation for this had been, but I think if I hadn't intervened, Nina would have hit the other patient.

All of these incidents emphasize the point made in the earlier story of Marilyn. Being around persons whom you perceive as confused isn't very reassuring if you're trying to get well yourself.

BB: Whatever the cause, the individual who is psychotic behaves in a way that seems strange to others or is unable to communicate coherently often is frightening to people in the setting. I think how staff respond to the confused person is very important. Clients and patients look at staff strategies and often model after them. If it is unclear to the patient or client group what strategies the staff are using, that can be quite distressing. If, for example, staff seem to be ignoring confused or psychotic behavior because they see it as innocuous, or they are being careful to reinforce only appropriate behavior, the patient group might misinterpret that to mean that staff are unaware of what's going on or that staff are incompetent. Sometimes treatment staff need to sit down with the patient group and describe specific strategies they are following or give the patient group some information and guidelines as to what they can do to cope with this behavior. I've been struck many times with how tolerant and supportive clients can be with each other when they have a means to understand behavior and some simple tools to deal with it. At times, clear-thinking clients will "buddy up" with their more confused peers, and we're able to make good use of that in the occupational therapy setting. But that's not always the case. I've also seen individuals and entire patient groups become quite insistent: they want a particular resident or group member to be removed from the setting. Some of these same issues come up when families have to deal with confused or inappropriate behavior of family members at home.

References

Kaplan, H., Sadock, B., & Grebb, J. (1994). *Kaplan and Sadock's synopsis of psychiatry* (7th ed.). Baltimore: Williams and Wilkins.

Kaplan, K. (1988). *Directive group therapy.* Thorofare, NJ: SLACK Inc.

Kielhofner, G. (1985). *A model of human occupation*. Baltimore: Williams and Wilkins.

Kielhofner, G. (1992). *Conceptual foundations of occupational therapy.* Philadelphia: F.A. Davis.

CHAPTER 6

Aggressive Behavior

KEY TOPICS

- Threatening behavior
- Adolescence
- Conduct disorder
- Safety
- Therapeutic milieu

Initial Comments

We now turn our attention to an encounter in which the therapist feels frightened. In this instance, the threat to safety is compelling. While the individual described in the story does not seem confused, the degree of his ability for self-control is in question. This story has much in common with the one in Chapter 5 in how the occupational therapist's response, again calm and consistent, is described. The therapeutic environment as depicted in this story does not seem as securely structured as the one in the preceding story of Kathy, and the reader may want to consider how the milieu could have been better organized to prevent the event that followed, or if it could.

Conduct Disorder

The central figure in this story is a 17-year-old young man diagnosed with conduct disorder with suicidal ideation. Conduct disorder is a diagnosis specific to childhood and adolescence. It is applied to persons over 18 only if their behavior does not meet the criteria established for antisocial personality disorder (Kaplan, Sadock, & Grebb, 1994, p. 1071). Conduct disorder is characterized by behavior that fails to meet age-appropriate social norms of conduct. There are two major subtypes of conduct disorder classified according to age of onset: childhood onset type (onset before age 10) and adolescent onset type (no conduct problems before the age of 10). The behavior of youths with this disorder includes aggression to people and animals, destruction of property, deceitfulness or theft, or serious violations regarding rules at home or school. Persistent truancy, hostile and defiant behavior toward adults, lying, vandalism, early sexual activity, and the use of tobacco, liquor, and drugs are all common with this disorder, and these youths make little effort to conceal their behavior. Suicidal thoughts and behavior are also common in this disorder. The *DSM-IV* (American Psychiatric Association, 1994) identifies levels of severity of the disorder, ranging from mild (e.g., few conduct problems causing minor harm) to severe (many behavior problems causing much harm) (Kaplan et al., 1994, p. 1071).

A variety of social, emotional, and biological factors are believed to contribute to this disorder, but none can be singled out. Children raised where there has been inconsistent parenting, abuse, or negligence may be more prone to this disorder. The coexistence of attention deficit/hyperactivity disorder and blood serotonin abnormalities suggests a possible central nervous system link. Temperament and personality variables in the child that make a poor fit with parenting needs and styles may also be contributory (Kaplan et al., 1994, p. 1072).

Intervention

Intervention with conduct disorder is often multi-pronged, with efforts made toward improving parenting, social and living conditions, and helping classroom teachers to respond to behavior (Kolko, 1992). Structured intervention programs often employ behaviorally oriented approaches, with consistent rules, expectations, and consequences for behavior. Youths with conduct disorder also may profit from learning problem-solving skills, since some of their behavior seems to result from ineffective coping with daily tasks (Kolko, 1992). The more severe the identified behavior(s), and the longer the conduct disorder has been going on, the more difficult it is to treat. Those with severe conduct disorder in youth are more vulnerable to other disorders in adulthood, including mood and substance-related disorders. A recent report, which perhaps is somewhat surprising, indicates that although assaultive behavior in childhood and parent criminality is predictive of imprisonment in adulthood, the diagnosis of conduct disorder per se is not correlated with incarceration (Kaplan et al., 1994, p. 1074).

"Frankie" Narrated by Mary E. Conrad, MBA, OTR/L

My patient, whom I'll call Frankie, was an angry-appearing 17-year-old young man. He was about 5′8″ and had a muscular build. Frankie was an inpatient in the treatment center where I worked, the psychiatric wing of a general hospital. Most of the inpatients had a relatively long treatment stay, although it varied from 1 to 2 weeks to several months depending on the situation. Frankie was quite belligerent, and had been unsuccessful in high school and at any attempted employments because he would sooner or later antagonize those in authority. Though Frankie pushed limits and was verbally aggressive, there was no indication in his history that he had ever harmed anyone. I had some adolescents I saw as a group, but I chose to see Frankie in a group of young adults, as they seemed to have more in common with Frankie than did the adolescents. Because Frankie used a lot of bravado, I also was concerned about the influence he might have on the adolescents and I felt he might make less of an impression on a slightly more mature patient group.

The day Frankie came into the clinic, I was working with a group of adults, although not those in his treatment group. The patients in the group were working on various projects of their own choosing. I noticed Frankie walk into the clinic and wondered to myself, "What's he doing here now? It's not time for his group," but I got distracted by a patient who called me over to ask for help. There was a knife lying on one of the work tables, which had just been used to trim up some leather. Very quickly, Frankie picked up the knife and walked behind me and said, "You know, I could cut your throat." I responded very quietly, "I know you could, but that's not what that knife is intended for. I want you to put it on the table." I repeated to him several times, "Put the knife on the table," in a slow, measured voice. Finally, he put it down and ran out of the clinic. Though I think I had been pretty calm and my voice was steady while this was going on, I immediately began to shake. The patient group who had witnessed his threat fell apart. Some started to cry; one woman had an epileptic seizure. I alerted the nursing staff back on the unit about what had occurred and they mobilized to secure Frankie. I also asked for nursing assistance to help the woman who had the seizure. My biggest concern quickly became members of the patient group who obviously were very frightened and needed to talk about what had happened, which we did.

I tried to think afterward about what I could have done to be in a less vulnerable position. There were several things to consider. For instance, we occasionally had hostile or combative patients in the hospital, but usually they were not allowed to come to occupational therapy if they were believed dangerous. Occasionally, a patient would be on a "hold and treat" and come to therapy with a police escort, but Frankie was not one of these people. The occupational therapy clinic was in a space set off from the nursing unit, but I ordinarily had a male industrial arts teacher using the clinic at the same time that I did. It just happened that on this day, he had not come into work. The treatment staff overall was not as careful as it might have been about ensuring that a staff member was never alone with the patient group. The staff often used occupational therapy time to do paperwork back on the unit, but then, we had not had an incident like this before. Maybe we had become lax. If I had known Frankie was a threat, I could have requested that he have an aide stay with him or that he be kept back on the unit, but I hadn't recognized the need. We did have an intercom system, but the speaker was in the office portion of the clinic, and not anywhere near where we were standing. Besides, making a quick move to reach the intercom wouldn't have been a very good idea.

I think much of what Frankie was doing was designed to impress the rest of the patients, but I'm not sure. The way he ran out of the clinic suggests that he got as frightened as we did. I've told students this story and always emphasize that this isn't typical of my experiences working in psychiatry, but it's probably the most scared I've ever been.

Discussion Questions

1. Have you ever been in a situation where a patient or client, child or adult, has threatened or intimidated you or another person? Describe how you or another person responded in the situation.
2. Discuss the scenario described in this narrative in terms of behavior management and safety. Given your limited information, what changes would you propose regarding policy or structure at this setting?
    a. What specific safety policies and procedures exist to manage client behavior in settings with which you are acquainted?
    b. In what ways are the previously identified policies similar or different? What might account for these variations?
3. If you were the therapist in this story, what would need to occur for you to feel safe with Frankie in your group in the future, or do you imagine that you could never feel safe with him?
4. Using your knowledge of conduct disorder, identify some strategies that the occupational therapist might use to manage Frankie's behavior.
5. If you had been the therapist narrating this story, and Frankie returned to your patient group (with appropriate supervision), what, if anything, would you like to say to him?
6. We learn that the patients who witnessed this incident were very distressed by it. Put yourself in the place of one of these patients. What might be your feelings or concerns?
7. What do you think the staff and/or the occupational therapist need to do to follow up with the patient group and help them again feel secure in this setting?
8. The narrator chose to have Frankie in a group of young adults rather than adolescents.
    a. What activities have you seen used within adolescent treatment groups? Young adult treatment groups?

b. In what ways might the therapeutic approach taken within an adolescent group be similar to or different from that taken when working with a group of young adults?

c. Which level therapy group do you believe represents the most appropriate level for Frankie: adolescent or adult?

Impressions

BB: An incident like this is often a wake-up call for staff to look at their policies and procedures and reevaluate how better to ensure safety. I've expressed my bias, which is that you can't focus on therapy in an environment where you are anxious regarding your safety—my priority is always safety. A concern raised by some of our students doing volunteer work and fieldwork in the community is that at certain centers there are protocols that, in students' perception, permit clients to attend therapy even when they are very volatile because of priorities given to the client's right to service. This has been described for school and nonschool settings. This, for me, represents something that needs to be considered very carefully. It may represent a swing in the pendulum from years ago when patients and clients (youth and adult) frequently were restricted from therapy as a consequence of undesirable behavior.

Even in the most structured and secured environments, the unexpected can happen, and it sounds like the narrating therapist responded just as she needed to. I've seen many instances where a staff person, whether it's a nurse, an aide, or a therapist, has managed a crisis by being very calm. You don't want to startle or threaten a person in Frankie's state.

We don't learn what ultimately happened to Frankie, or how staff responded to him around this incident. His behavior suggested a loss of judgment and control, and, in addition to being concerned about his being a danger to others, the suicide risk for him could also increase. I suspect that Frankie wouldn't feel safe if he perceives that staff are not effectively in charge. I wonder how our storyteller felt when she again had Frankie in the treatment group, assuming that happened.

MAB: When reflecting on my clinical experience, I recall few times when I felt unsafe. I believe that there is a need for safety protocol in all settings. For example, I have worked in settings where policy states that when treating patients in their room, the door should remain open. When treating patients with a history of aggression, staff should be aware of those conditions that trigger aggression, have a plan for supervising the patient, and have an emergency system for communication in place. I believe therapists also should consider the option of not treating a patient when they are afraid or the patient is upset or angry. As you see, my emphasis is on prevention. However, the unexpected occurs, as evidenced in the story of Frankie. In such an event, team members must have the opportunity to discuss the event and their fears afterward, and then revise their plan for behavior management. The therapist could then modify his or her occupational therapy treatment sessions accordingly.

References

American Psychiatric Association. (1994). *Diagnostic and statistical manual of mental disorders* (4th ed.). Washington, DC: Author.

Kaplan, H., Sadock, B., & Grebb, J. (1994). *Kaplan and Sadock's synopsis of psychiatry* (7th ed.). Baltimore: Williams and Wilkins.

Kolko, D. (1992). Conduct disorder. In V.B. Van Hasselt & D. Kolko (Eds.), *Inpatient behavior therapy for children and adolescents* (pp. 205-237). New York: Plenum Press.

CHAPTER 7

Quality of Life

KEY TOPICS

- The wish to die
- Manipulation
- Quality of life
- Adult development issues
- Integrity versus despair
- Chronic pain
- Pain management
- Caretaking
- Educating staff

Initial Comments

Some comments frequently heard when working with adolescents and adults, in acute and long-term care and within a variety of treatment and nontraditional settings, express the idea, "I wish I could just lie down and die" or "never wake up," "I'd be better off dead," or "My family would be better off without me."

As we discuss in another text (Bruce & Borg, 1993), it is believed normal for a person at some time to consider what it would be like to die, and to consider the possibility of taking his or her own life. That is not the same as being actively suicidal, which suggests a strong attraction to the idea of suicide as a solution to the problems of one's suffering or hopelessness. As occupational therapists, we want to clarify whether or not an individual who comments that he or she wants to die is suicidal. We may be in a position where we need to ask whether or not the person has a suicide plan, or help caregivers determine the risk for suicide in other ways. This allows care providers to intervene as needed. Often, however, these expressions actually communicate hopelessness and a giving up on life. Hearing people verbalize their wish to die can be disarming and stir our own feelings as we try to listen and respond without minimizing the individual's feelings.

In this chapter, we present three separate stories, with Discussion Questions and Impressions following each story. The main figure in each of the narratives makes a comment about perhaps being better off dead, which reflects his or her need to have a say in his or her life and to attain a desired quality of life.

The clients in all of our stories are individuals who have had a high profile in the community and have been able, in the past, to take charge. These are stories about struggling to cope with physical pain and physical decline while maintaining a sense of integrity and worth.

Linking Developmental Tenets

In the first and third of our next three narratives, one is reminded of the life stages described by Erikson (1959). Both of the central figures are older adults, one in his 70s and the other 93. According to Erikson, they are at a stage in life where they must accept physical decline, redirect energy into new channels, and develop a point of view about death—all toward the goal of achieving a sense of integrity and self-worth rather than despair (Erikson, 1959; Erikson, Erikson, & Kivnik, 1986). It is a time in life, according to Erikson (1959), Jung (1933), and other developmentalists (Gould, 1972, 1978; Levinson, 1980; Neugarten 1964, 1979) when introspection and reminiscence are important activities.

Bernice Neugarten (1979) writes that the older person must work out "a balance between the losses and the victories" (p. 893). For occupational therapists, these losses and victories play out in the everyday activities of life. Often, old standards of performance cannot be met and accomplishments are measured by new yardsticks. Balancing losses with victories is not exclusive to older age, however. A goal of therapy in all three stories is to help each client accept limitations while finding meaning in life. Trying to understand the client's lifestyle and his or her particular ways of participating in the family and social culture becomes an important part of the therapy process. If this can be accomplished and the individual meets personal challenges in a way consistent with his or her lifestyle, the person achieves a sense of mastery and becomes better able to deal with future challenges. One theme that emerges in all of the narratives is the importance of everyday activities in maintaining dignity and self-respect, something we see over and over throughout the book.

Introduction to "Mr. Callahan"

Our first story is about a man in his 70s who has experienced many losses and deals with chronic pain. It seems consistent with what we know about the developmental tasks of older age that he might ask himself, "Is it worth going on?" But when he poses this question to the therapist, important ethical issues are crystallized as she considers how best to respond.

"Mr. Callahan" Narrated by Barbara Borg, MA, OTR

Mr. Callahan came from a family with a long history of wealth and influence in the East. By his own account, he had gone through two fortunes, not because of excessive spending on his part, but due to the vicissitudes of an unpredictable stock market. He seemed an exceptionally bright and articulate man who in the past had a great deal of influence in business and within his church and community. He had the assistance of hired help throughout his life, and expected exemplary service. Now, many years later, he was a widower in his early 70s, wiry and quite strong from a lifetime of daily, rigorous exercise. One of the routines which he still did daily was to spend 30 minutes climbing and descending the stairs of his 12-story residence.

Mr. Callahan had peripheral vascular disease which had resulted in severe pain in his right arm. The pain required his taking several strong pain medications that left his speech slurred and his thoughts unclear on many days. According to his medical history he was also "legally blind," a phrase I mistakenly understood to mean he couldn't see anything but shadows or outlines.

When I first met Mr. Callahan, he had just come home from surgery to remove a blood clot in his right axilla. He looked thin and drawn, and told me that he had lost almost 25 pounds. His demeanor was stern and guarded. Sometime during our first visit, I asked about his eyesight, and he told me flatly that he was "blind." It was soon after that I surmised that he had some vision, although I remained uncertain about the extent to which he could perceive detail.

The referral to occupatioanl therapy came about, in part, because he was not using his right hand or arm in any activities. The right hand was so sensitive to touch and so cold that he frequently kept it covered by a heavy sock. His hand was also showing the beginning signs of flexor contracture. Although previous therapists had fitted him with resting splints, he adamantly refused to wear them.

The nurse who first asked me to see Mr. Callahan was concerned about his depression, and asked me to help her assess his suicide risk. He and I talked about this on a number of occasions; most often he couched this by saying that he felt that his quality of life was such that he didn't care to go on, though he wasn't ready to take his own life. "Do you think it's morally wrong to kill yourself?" he asked one day. I equivocated and responded that this was a personal question we each had to decide for ourselves—not as much of a nonanswer as I might have initially thought. He pondered aloud about his own quality of life. The pain in his right hand was constant and kept him from paying attention to much else; he knew he wasn't communicating clearly which frustrated and embarrassed him. Although he could read with the assistance of technology that projected words from his books onto a big-screen television, he felt he couldn't concentrate on reading—an activity he had formerly enjoyed. He couldn't see, as he said, "worth a damn." Since he could barely tolerate using his right arm and hand or have them touched, and was right hand dominant, he was awkward in all of his self-care tasks including dressing, bathing, and eating. This man, who had been a major player in the stock exchange, now dribbled food on his white sport shirts.

Mr. Callahan reminded me of many others I had met who seemed to find the worst consequence of their illness to be the loss of control and dignity. While he didn't actively prepare for it, suicide represented one way to have control over his own life. He told me once that the only reason he hadn't killed himself was because he knew his family would be "so upset."

Because Mr. Callahan expressed concern about appearing messy when he ate with his peers in the dining room, one of the first things we arranged was for me to be his guest at lunch. I hoped that I might observe and give him some pointers on simple adaptations that would facilitate handling food. There, he and his tablemates talked about a book that two at the table were reading, *Let Me Die Before I Wake: Hemlock's Book of Self-Deliverance* (Humphry, 1987), a book that gave instructions on how to commit suicide. I was particularly struck by how the group lowered their voices so no one outside their group could hear what they were talking about.

In addition to supporting Mr. Callahan during his depression and trying to help him regain some control in his everyday activities, I worked with him on pain management in collaboration with physical therapy. He had been given a TENS unit intended to block the conduction of painful nerve impulses. We experimented with having Mr. Callahan use his right arm and hand in functional activities like making a sandwich or combing his hair, either with the unit on or following its use. Unexpectedly, pain management ceased to be a goal.

From the time I first met Mr. Callahan, he had a small closed sore on his right thumb—nothing more, it seemed, than a roughened, red spot. As with people who have diabetes or other peripheral vascular disease, this sore healed slowly and remained unchanged for many weeks. Then, in a matter of days, it started to redden and ooze, and within a week a staph infection was identified. With minimal circulation to the hand, the infection worsened. His physician advised Mr. Callahan that the decision was his, but that if his antibiotics didn't start having an effect, his life would be in danger if he didn't allow the hand to be amputated. His family gathered more information, while Mr. Callahan asked me and other caregivers, "Should I wait, or have the hand taken?" Sensing how important it was that he feel some control, yet wanting to communicate my care for him, I squeezed his left hand and could only say, "John, remember, you are more than a hand." It was 8 more days before he gave the go-ahead and the arm and hand were removed just below the elbow.

The stump healed quickly, and for the first time in over a year, the pain in his arm abated. He was able to discontinue his pain medication within 2 weeks of his surgery, and his cognition cleared. Within a month, he had gained 15 pounds and began to talk again about the quality of his life, But this time, he maintained that his life had some quality. "You know," he said, "when you're in constant pain it takes all your energy. You can't think of anything else. You have no life."

Now my visits were to help him prepare the stump for an eventual prosthesis. He couldn't close his right elbow past 90 degrees, nor could he pronate it or supinate it. I called his prosthetist to ask what might be causing the tightness. He answered that some surgeons are not thinking about prosthetics when they repair an arm, and they often pull the tendons so tight so as to prohibit full motion. I relayed this to Mr. Callahan, who did not seem particularly concerned. "I don't really care if I can use the darn thing," he said. "A prosthesis will just look better." One day he said, "Tell your students when people are sick, they are sick mentally, too, and you have to help them with that—that's the real battle." As we prepared for the end of my visits, Mr. Callahan told me that he appreciated that I always looked him in the eyes when I talked to him.

Discussion Questions

1. Characterize the client-therapist relationship in the story of Mr. Callahan.
2. What did you learn from this narrative?
3. Why do you believe Mr. Callahan might have led the therapist to believe he was totally blind when he wasn't?
4. How important is it to you that you have control in your own life?
   a. Do you think yours would be a life of quality if you couldn't exert control to the extent you do now?
   b. In what areas would you be willing to give up control?
5. Put yourself in the therapist's place and consider what your response would be if a client asked, "Is it morally wrong to kill yourself?" Reflect carefully on what your response communicates.
6. If a client such as Mr. Callahan told you he or she had decided to take his or her own life, how would you feel? What would you do?
7. What is the legal definition of "legally blind"?
   a. Based upon this definition, what would you consider when you evaluate and treat individuals who have visual impairments?
   b. What services or resources are you aware of in your community for helping persons who have impaired vision?
8. Have you witnessed or been directly involved with clients who have chosen not to follow recommended adaptations to perform activities of daily living (ADL) or other occupations?
   a. Describe what you perceived as being responsible for their hesitation.
   b. What do you believe would have been a helpful response by the therapist?

Impressions

BB: Mr. Callahan was my client. As I reread his story and have some distance from it, it reminds me a bit of a teeter-totter. When I first met him, the losses experienced by Mr. Callahan were not balanced by the victories. It was when his hand and lower arm were amputated and his pain subsided that the balance seemed to change, and the story changed. He became much healthier physically and again had an emotional reserve. I believe he made an important reaffirmation during the course of talking about his own possible suicide. In his own estimation he had been "mentally sick," which I suspect for him had to do with not being certain if he was going to meet life head-on any longer, or just let himself slip away.

Bernice Neugarten, whom we cite in our Initial Comments, tells us that it is important for older adults to be able to pass on their wisdom. Mr. Callahan knew that I was teaching at Colorado State when I was his therapist. His comment, "Tell your students when people are sick, they are sick mentally, too, and you have to help them with that...," is an example of wisdom sharing. There was another instance that I didn't include in the story but would like to relate here. Throughout my time with Mr. Callahan, I believed him to be blind, and I was very aware of wanting to use all possible active listening skills when talking with him. This included looking into his eyes, although I didn't believe he could see where I was looking. At our last therapy session, as we were saying "Goodbye," Mr. Callahan said that he liked that I looked him in the eyes when we talked, and he said, "Tell your students that eye contact is important." I think he was enjoying teasing me and letting me know that he could see more than what I had thought. Anyway, now I've passed that along.

At the time I was seeing Mr. Callahan, one of the things that especially impressed me was how many of his peers thoughtfully weighed the pros and cons of taking their own lives, and it was not necessarily those who were in poor health or who appeared depressed. Rather, it included relatively healthy individuals who were accustomed to living a quality of life and managing their own affairs. They wanted to know that, should their health or abilities take a sharp decline, they would have a way out. I believe that they wanted to live life on their own terms, and that included determining when they'd had enough.

MAB: I was especially struck by this patient's statement, "When you're in constant pain...you have no life." I have heard this comment frequently from clients of all ages who have chronic pain. I've dealt with similar treatment issues as those described in this story, including responding to depression and anger, finding ways to manage pain, and helping people determine how they can "have a life." Unlike with Mr. Callahan, none of my clients had an instant cure, so to speak.

The way people can manage everyday tasks has a huge effect on their quality of life. Just as with Mr. Callahan, for example, I've had clients and their families who were concerned about messy eating habits. It prevents many of these individuals from eating out in the community and from socializing around meals. This takes much of the pleasure from life. Although I've made some suggestions that involved the use of adaptive equipment, many clients adamantly refuse adaptive equipment or are only willing to use it at home.

Introduction to "Anita"

The woman described below lives with chronic pain, and, like "Mr. Callahan," has wondered, "Is it worth going on?" Anita must deal with loss and the prospect of chronic pain as a woman in middle, rather than late, life.

"Anita" Narrated by Mary Ann Bruce, MS, OTR

Anita, a woman in her early 40s, was not my patient. Rather, I was asked by her neuropsychologist to consult with him regarding the dilemmas he felt in trying to help her. I had had many informal chats with Anita as she and one of my patients shared gym space, and in some ways I felt she and I had already had some rapport. Since Anita had no insurance coverage for occupational therapy, I suggested to her that she and I have lunch if she was in agreement. She agreed enthusiastically, but verbalized concern that she wouldn't be able to sit in one place for the 40 minutes she felt we'd need to eat out. I suggested that we meet at the hospital cafeteria where her standing would draw less attention. When we met for lunch, she immediately said, "This is a treat for me. It's the first time I've eaten out in a couple of years. I'm sorry I can't take you out to...(a popular and expensive local restaurant)." She told me that she had been managing pain for several years due to a spinal abscess and subsequent surgeries. She was unable to sit for more than 10 minutes. Hers was a story of multiple losses: she had lost her position in the art community, her spouse (who could not cope with the lifestyle changes her condition had brought about), many friends who were uncomfortable being around her, her business which she could no longer manage, and her independent lifestyle and feelings of effectiveness. She described feeling that there was nothing left that she could do, and she wondered aloud, "Is life worth living?"

I talked to Anita about time management strategies and breaking activities up into small units. Also, rather than developing totally new interests, I proposed that she set a small, achievable goal that allowed her to continue with what she enjoyed, which for her was art. I gave her several examples of what might be reasonable, small goals. The lunch hour went much too quickly, but Anita said she felt she had a start and "hope." She agreed to keep me informed of her decisions and activities, and I told her I would share my recommendations with her psychologist. Over the next several months, I conversed informally with Anita. As she discovered that there were activities she could accomplish in 10-minute increments, she started feeling more empowered. Then she generated her own ideas about how she could reposition herself physically to improve her own comfort, and how to become reinvolved in her community and with the activities that she had enjoyed. Art was her passion, and she decided to contact her network of colleagues and propose some roles that she could assume from her home. Within a brief time, she became a volunteer consultant on several local museum boards. Her appearance also was important to her, and she arranged to have a shopping consultant obtain clothes for her at a favorite department store. From this we see how everyday activities and the pursuit of personal interests empowered this individual, and helped her build confidence that she would be able to problem solve and live a quality life.

Discussion Questions

1. What perceptions or assumptions does Anita appear to have that have led her to wonder if life is worth living?
2. Do you believe that people approach the question "Is life worth living?" differently depending on their age and place in the life span?
3. What factors do you believe contribute to the positive outcome of this story?
4. As described in this story, the narrator was not engaged in occupational therapy intervention with this woman. If you had been this woman's occupational therapist, what would have been your approach in helping Anita manage chronic pain?
   a. What will be the theoretical basis for this approach?
   b. How would you incorporate previous activity interests?
   c. How would you incorporate principles related to energy conservation? Biomechanics?
5. Do you believe that the narrating therapist was "giving away" her services? How would you have handled this request for consultation?
6. The literature is steeped in the mandate to "empower" our clients. What does this mean to you?

Impressions

BB: It seems to me that the story for this woman changes when she can start to see her situation through your eyes—at that point, she states that she has "hope." For all we know, others might have suggested the kind of approach you described, where she would break up her activities into small units, but it seemed that during your lunch meeting something opened up for her. This also is a story about a woman who has resources and a viable support system. The social and physical environment seem to be vital factors in the story's outcome.

MAB: This story raises another concern. On occasion, I have consulted with clients or other professionals treating clients not referred to occupational therapy and then wondered if I was giving away my services. I tend to help when needed. However, recent experiences have made me consider all of my options, which might include a one time consult for evaluation or to share information with another professional expecting that the patient will be referred to occupational therapy for services. Still, I have mixed feelings, particularly because I often see other professionals incorporating what looks like occupational therapy into their intervention as they try to meet the expectation for functional outcomes.

Introduction to "Leave Me Alone"

Our next story begins with the central figure, a 93-year-old woman, saying, in essence, "I wish you'd let me die." In contrast to the earlier story of Mr. Callahan, the therapist doesn't respond philosophically, but gives a matter-of-fact response.

As you read this next account, we ask you to think not only about the response given to the patient's comments that she'd like to be left alone to die, but also to the amount of control that the occupational therapist gives the patient overall in their interaction. As the story evolves, the narrator cites the term "manipulative," a term that is often applied when describing clients and patients. Reflect on what this word really means, and how occupational therapists can respond best in this kind of situation.

"Leave Me Alone" (Anonymous)

Once I was asked to treat a debilitated 93-year-old woman who was recovering from a hip fracture. On my very first meeting with her, she said, "I wish you'd just leave me alone and let me lie here and die." She was obviously very frustrated with her slow recovery and was refusing many of the therapists' and staff's efforts. I tried to help her see that lying in bed would not necessarily increase the likelihood she would die, at least not comfortably. I explained that if she stayed in bed, her remaining days could bring more discomfort due to skin breakdown and the likelihood of decubiti. But I also listened to and let her reminisce. I spent about 10 to 15 minutes sitting with her as she told me about life as the spouse of a prominent attorney and her outrage at the "goings on" of recent televised court hearings. After that, she agreed to do her basic ADL tasks, upper body exercises, and to practice bed mobility.

We got into a routine. In several subsequent sessions, I would use the first part of the session to listen to the same or very similar stories when I went to work with her on her daily ADLs. Then she was able to turn her attention to our therapy tasks. Some of the therapists in this setting felt that this patient was manipulative and should not be allowed to control the treatment session in this manner. I did not bring to her attention that she had told me these stories before. For a number of reasons, I chose to see her for her ADLs after lunch. She had indicated that she liked to sleep late, didn't want to be interrupted during the news, and preferred to do hygiene after eating lunch and before she went to afternoon physical therapy and then rested. Until I started working in this facility, I would have assumed that basic ADL tasks had to be done in the morning. One of my problems when working with this woman was that if the communication was not clear to the certified nursing assistants (CNAs) that I was coming, a CNA would arrive early in the morning and do her ADLs for her. He or she would bathe and dress her without having her help because it was faster for the CNA.

Over the next month in which I worked with her, I saw her cooperate more and more with occupational and physical therapy, and she spent an increased amount of time out of bed. Gradually she got stronger, and was able to do her basic ADLs while sitting, and was able to mobilize with a walker. She eventually returned home, which for her was an apartment in the same retirement community, although she needed daily help and supervision.

Discussion Questions

1. What did you learn from this story?
2. Think about the therapist's response to the patient's request that she be "left alone to die." The therapist responded by pointing out that the patient's refusal to cooperate might result in more discomfort and decubiti. Are you comfortable with this response? Why or why not?
3. Describe other strategies for responding to this patient's initial resistance to treatment.
4. In addition to conversation, what treatment activities can be used to facilitate life review?
5. If part or all of a treatment session were used to allow a client to engage in reminiscence or life review, how would you document and charge for this part of the therapy process?
6. Do you think the patient in this story was given too much control regarding scheduling and the particulars of her treatment?
    a. Was the therapist being manipulated? Support your position and suggest an alternative approach if you think one is called for.
    b. Identify your theoretical frame of reference as you describe how you would have liked to see the therapist interact with this patient.
7. Identify the information that you believe needs to be shared with CNAs in this story to have their support for achieving this resident's goals.
8. Describe some methods the occupational therapist could use to maintain ongoing communication or education with the CNAs or nurses' aides dealing with patient care.
9. In what ways do you think perceptions and values relative to a client's age or particular disability influence caregiving? Have you seen instances where this varied, specific to cultural or family values?
10. Describe instances when you have struggled with issues around wanting to do more for a client, or feeling that you (or others) were doing too much for a client during self-care or in the context of other daily activities.

CHAPTER 8

Normal Development

KEY TOPICS

- Client expectations
- Therapist as expert
- Traumatic brain injury
- Emotional changes in acquired brain impairment
- Holism
- Developmental issues with the younger client
- Parent concerns
- Medical ethics

Initial Comments

The following narrative centers on an adolescent's feelings that he has no say in what occurs in therapy. His comments suggest an underlying belief that as a young person he should do whatever is instructed by the therapist because the therapist is the authority, and doing what she says is the way to get well. In giving him an increased say in decisions, the narrator's response takes into account this young man's developmental needs for independence and increased self-confidence. As she thinks about her responses to this adolescent, the narrating therapist reflects on other instances in which patients/clients and their families have expected her to behave as the boss or expert, and have been critical when she tried to include them in the decision-making process. There are many dimensions to this story. As you read, try to recall what it was like to be 15 years old, and what you needed from adults and your peers at that time. We also would like you to recall personal medical or therapy situations in which it was especially important for you to trust that you were in the hands of experts who would help you regain health.

Developmental Issues

The main person in our narrative is 15 years old. According to developmental theory, beginning at birth and with each life period or stage the person has specific issues and challenges that must be mastered. New ways of thinking and responding at each stage represent new forms of adaptation. For our 15-year-old, that is a time in life when he should be becoming more independent, even rebellious, questioning authority, and separating more from his family. It is a time when peer relationships are very important, including comfortable relationships with the opposite sex, and when he needs to be taking an increasing amount of responsibility for decision making. As we read, circumstances intervene that significantly impede this young man's ability for these developmental challenges.

Jeff in this story, Nathan in Chapter 9's story, and several individuals in upcoming narratives have had traumatic brain injury (TBI). Their stories bring to life the comments we make here. All of these stories illustrate the interplay of psychosocial, neurological, and physical components within the context of an environment that creates expectations and provides support. Understandably, the way mind-body-spirit responds often reflects previous coping mechanisms and personal style. Rather than describe emotional responses in detail through our didactic information, our goal throughout the text is to illustrate emotional issues within the context of our stories. We would, however, like to make a few additional comments.

Acquired Brain Impairments, Emotions, and Development

TBI is one of many acquired brain impairments, all of which significantly affect a person's "inner life," or cognition and emotions (Fine, 1993). The person afflicted with brain impairment most often copes with multiple changes and losses in their lifestyle and life roles, in the way they can play, participate in school, or work; within personal relationships; and as related to diverse physical, emotional, cognitive, and other functional skills. Not only are there losses in abilities and resources, there are frequently increased demands placed on the client and the family by what Fine (1993) aptly refers to as the "interminable medical procedures" (p. 7) that often accompany brain trauma. Brain injury is much like other conditions, among them stroke, multiple sclerosis, Alzheimer's disease and other dementias, schizophrenia, depression, and bipolar disorder, in which there are consistent or recurring disruptions in the ability to process and act upon information in a cogent way. Whatever their genesis, cognitive impairments place tremendous stress on clients, their families, and close associates. With brain impairments, visions of oneself and of one's own (and the family's) future change.

Emotional responses may be specific to the site of central nervous system injury or lesion (e.g., to arousal centers), may be the result of more diffuse central nervous system disruption, or may result from the emotional strain of dealing with so many changes coming from so many directions. The rehabilitation process is often long and intense. Individuals find themselves in unfamiliar environments and engaged in tasks that may be perceived as strange or disconnected. Both children and adults may become depressed and anxious, feel lonely and vulnerable, and feel as if they have little control. They frequently experience a decreased sense of self-worth and identity. These emotional/cognitive changes and alterations in self-perception influence their sense of physical well-being, the ability to initiate and regulate motivated behavior, and the ability to judge, feel, and think about one's place in the world. These inner life factors also impact interests and values, management of stress, and future coping abilities. Ultimately, emotional factors will support or interfere with adaptation (Fine, 1990, 1993). If the client is a youth who also is handling the physical and emotional changes that go along with adolescence, has altered perceptions of himself or herself as a soon-to-be adult, and has developmental needs to strike out on his or her own, the mix of issues becomes very complex.

Holistic Practice

The reader is referred to a compelling endorsement by Fine (1990, 1993) of holistically based practice of occupational therapy as a means to respond to the multiple and dynamic sequelae associated with cognitive impairments. The holistic model frames the adaptive process by appreciating that each person and environmental context is unique. It is a transactional model in that it looks at the ongoing give and take between all of the developmental domains (biological, emotional, cognitive, and interpersonal) as well those making up the environment (family, community, and society at large) (Cicchetti, Rogosch, & Toth, 1994, p. 132; Fine, 1993). One's place in the life span helps shape his or her expectations, values, and resources.

A holistic model demands that we as therapists not view emotions as something "out there" to be managed by our peers working in the so-called "psychosocial area." Challenging all occupational therapists to address clients' and families' emotional needs, Fine (1993) writes:

> *The psychosocial domain is everybody's business. It must not be disregarded as something irrelevant to your practice, disposed of because you think it won't be reimbursed, or dismissed because someone else on your team is expected to deal with it. The fact is, you can't discard it because it doesn't go away. It's omnipresent—to help you or to hinder you in your work with each individual. (p. 10)*

A holistic, transactional model helps us, as therapists, pay attention to the importance of the relationships between clients, caregivers, and significant others (Fine, 1993, p. 25). The occupational therapist works with families to support their adjustment to the role of caregiver, and with families, educators, and others to increase their understanding of disability and the adaptive process.

There is no single profile of the emotional response to TBI, whether we are considering young people or adults. As individuals learn to cope and adapt during therapy, emotional reactions vary. Some will struggle to maintain an optimistic outlook, and may have angry emotional outbursts or seem to feel defeated; others may seem cavalier or lethargic. In terms of the developmental process, adolescents would be expected to have the ability for empathy and to decenter, younger children might not. However, cognitive changes may compromise the ability of a child, adolescent, or adult to be empathic and consider the needs of others. Individuals may be impatient or irritable and withdraw socially. Others are outgoing and nondiscriminating in initiating social contact.

Trying to modulate emotional reactions can be very wearisome, especially in light of all the other demands being made on the person physically and cognitively. Individuals of all ages can become overwhelmed by stress and therapy demands.

As you read the upcoming stories in which brain impairment exists, think about where the client is in the life span. What developmentally linked expectation might he or she be facing? Pay attention to the thoughts and feelings that the main individuals seem to be experiencing. How do these emotions affect the person's sense of self, the therapeutic and family relationships, and the use and success of specific intervention strategies?

"Jeff" Narrated by Mary Ann Bruce, MS, OTR

This story is about a young man, Jeff, who was 15 years old when I first met him. He had been a very popular high school sophomore—a youngster who his peers looked up to. Then he experienced a traumatic head injury from a skateboard accident. While in a coma, he was diagnosed with leukemia. Jeff had multiple physical and neurological symptoms and impairments, as well as emotional and behavior responses to address in treatment.

I began working with Jeff in a home care program following approximately 1 year of hospitalization. Although he could get into the community, he had home-based rather than outpatient service at the insistence of his physician who was concerned about the risk of infection with Jeff. His home services included a school tutor, physical therapy, occupational therapy, speech therapy, vision therapy, and psychological counseling.

I worked with Jeff for about a year and a half. During that time our goals varied and included improving his balance, building his attention, increasing his ability for age-appropriate social interactions, and resuming a myriad of everyday tasks that had been a part of his life before his trauma and illness. A partial list of the activities that we used included: picking up in his room and making his bed, grooming and personal hygiene, preparing snacks and doing simple cooking, cleaning up in the kitchen, playing board and computer games, and performing activities designed to get him back into the community. When Jeff was first injured, his friends dropped by often to see him. Over time, however, their visits became less frequent and he had become quite socially isolated. When they did visit, his friends would tell him about their day, but he had little to say about his. He still slept a great deal and seldom watched television, so even talk about favorite television programs was difficult for him to participate in. Venturing into the community seemed vital to his resumption of normal adolescent activities, and I obtained his physician's permission to do this. One of our first activities, his mom's choice, was attending a high school football game. We also resumed the kinds of activities an adolescent would do (e.g., going to the mall to purchase Christmas cards for his mom, grandmother, and sister, then going back to the mall another day to have lunch). Throughout this process, I tried to involve his mother at an appropriate level, while encouraging her to let Jeff increase his independence.

One of the recurring problems I had in the early phase of intervention with this family was that when I tried to speak with his mother regarding recommendations or his progress, he consistently interrupted us. During the course of treatment he had become especially demanding of her attention, and didn't like to have his mother out of his sight.

One day after working with Jeff, he and I got to talking about his achievements in therapy and his feelings about rehabilitation. He identified that what he liked least about rehabilitation was that "you can't say 'no'." His response still causes me to think about his situation, as well as that of others with children and adults I have worked with in therapy. After giving it some thought, I suspected that I did communicate the expectation that he go along with whatever I said, but also that pressures came from within himself and from his family.

He had stated on numerous occasions, "The only way that I'll get better is to do what I'm supposed to do in therapy." This comment sounded a lot like what I had heard his mother say to him, when she would say that we (therapists) were going to help him get better. We were the experts, so to speak. I wondered if this positive expectation and the trust in the many health care providers who came into his home helped both him and his mother keep going. I know, too, that his mother had firm expectations for the client as well as his younger sister. Both young people seemed to respect their mom and appeared attuned to her challenges as a single parent. Although I had never heard her say it in these exact words, I sensed the expectation was "Do as you are told."

After thinking about how I wanted to respond, I indicated to Jeff that he was free to ask me why he was being given certain therapy tasks or to say "no," and we could talk about it. Another tactic I took was to include him more in the dialogues I had with his mother. When I needed to talk to his mother, I would say to Jeff, "I need to talk to your mom. Why don't you listen, too." I went from permitting him to listen to inviting him in. That seemed to work well in terms of his interrupting much less often.

I never did get into a lengthy discussion regarding who was in charge, or the value of therapy, or anything about my expertise. These issues didn't seem to be interfering with therapy or his progress. However, I became more conscious of giving Jeff a choice between two alternatives with specific expectations. In this instance, giving him choices seemed effective in responding to his emotional needs as well as increasing his sense of responsibility for the focus and direction of his own therapy. It made a better fit with his needs as an adolescent.

As therapy progressed, he began to initiate discussions regarding his treatment program and its focus. Sometimes he asked if I had a preference for the sequence of treatment activities, and sometimes he disagreed with my treatment plan and would propose an appropriate alternative. His mother also mentioned that he had begun to initiate discussions with her about how they would carry out treatment at home. She reported that she often would let him make decisions. As he continued to practice decision making, he began to generalize and expect other therapists to give him similar freedom. Not all of his therapists wanted him to make choices within their therapy sessions. In fact, some therapists suggested he had a behavior problem when he refused to cooperate with their treatment plans. These conflicting expectations were eventually discussed in a team meeting and guidelines were developed.

It's been almost a year since I worked with Jeff. Jeff now participates in a public high school program for 2 hours a day. It is a special program designed to meet the needs of students who are transitioning back into school. His program includes some academic coursework tailored to fit his abilities plus social activity. He continues to show improvement and there is hope that he eventually will be able to resume coursework within the regular class program, although not at the same grade level.

I knew I wanted to encourage Jeff to be more independent and to question what we were doing, and it was understandable that he might not be sure if doing that was permissible. But this interaction with Jeff reminds me of instances in which adult clients have seemed offended by being offered choices within their therapy, and have questioned my competence. On several occasions when I've asked clients to make decisions that would influence the course of their treatment, these clients have countered with comments such as "Isn't that (being the expert and making decisions) what I pay you for?"

Discussion Questions

1. Restate in your own words how you think Jeff feels within this narrative. How do these feelings seem to change?
   a. Put yourself in Jeff's place and describe how you think you might feel. What might your concerns be?
   b. Assume you had given up most of your former activities for more than a year. What activities would you, as a 15-year-old, have wanted to return to?
2. What might be your concerns as Jeff's parent? Prioritize these.
3. Have you ever been in a situation where you have counted on the medical expertise of others?
   a. Did you question or challenge the treatment that was recommended?
   b. How did you feel in the situation?
4. If you have observed instances of client noncompliance, to what did you attribute

this resistance? How could you respond to noncompliance?

5. How might therapists directly or indirectly pressure clients to participate or comply with therapy, or to not question what they are being asked to do?
6. How would you respond to this patient's comment that he "can't say 'no'"?
7. Assume that a client tells you, "You're the expert. Tell me what I can expect as an outcome of your therapy services."
   a. Identify what might be the motive in his or her making such a request.
   b. How might you respond?

Impressions

MAB: Jeff was my client and I wanted to include his story because it gives us an opportunity to reflect on some of the special challenges in applying a client-centered approach with adolescents. It also gives us an opportunity to discuss some of the different ways the therapist's authority can be viewed. On one occasion my client was a lawyer, a man in his late 40s, who had a large law practice and had been active in his family and the community. He had a cerebral vascular accident and made what seemed to be a good recovery. He had regained his speech and walked without noticeable impairment, but he felt less than perfect. Recognizing that he couldn't think as quickly on his feet, he decided not to go back into court situations. Thinking back, one of the things of which he was most critical was the change he saw in his signature when he signed checks and other important documents. With his therapy coming to an end, this client came to a weekly support group that I led. He expressed that he was dissatisfied with therapy services because we, as therapists, never could tell him what the end-product of our services would be. He knew we couldn't answer that exactly, but he wanted some odds or probabilities of certain functions returning. He indicated that as a lawyer, he was expected to tell people what they could expect for their money. And he asked us, "What am I getting for my money?"

A similar reaction came from a businessman I had to contact in my role as the case manager for another client. My client had worked for this man for more than 20 years and they both wanted my client to return to work. My client gave me permission to call his employer so I could determine exactly what his job entailed, so that we might be able to identify adaptations that would make it easier to resume employment. The first question his employer asked me was, "When will he be able to return to work?" When I responded that his doctor made the decision and that my responsibility was to identify the compatibility of his job expectations with his current function, he appeared irritated and said, in essence, that those of us in the health care field "...can be specific about your fee schedule, but not about what you can deliver." He added, "As a businessman, I tell my customers what they can expect for their money." This was compounded because this employer was contributing toward the client's medical bills. I could tell that he was frustrated, and, I suspected, had feelings about this before we'd spoken. I couldn't help but think he had a valid point.

BB: It seems to me that although Jeff is 15 years old, many of the early descriptions used in the narrative evoke the image of working with a young child; for instance, he doesn't want his mother "out of his sight," he's "demanding of attention," and wants to be able to say "no." As when working with children, many of the therapist exchanges seem to be between mother and therapist. No wonder he feels that he has little control. It almost seems that somewhere during your interaction with Jeff you recognize that he needs to be viewed more as an adult. The activities you describe sound very much like what a typical 15-year-old would do. As the mother of a 15-year-old, I know my son has a strong need to feel that what he does is by choice and not because he is being told what to do. I'd guess that Jeff has that same need, but it is a bit riskier for him to challenge you—after all, he depends on you and his other therapists so much. I don't know the extent of his cognitive impairment, but we know that many individuals seem to regress to earlier emotional levels of function when they deal with disease or traumatic events. As you pointed out earlier, when we're sick, we often like to be taken care of and have our needs met, and on some level that may be true for Jeff also. Or, he might vacillate between wanting to be independent and wanting to be taken care of. I believe that's normal for adolescents also. I think Jeff took a chance, and one that proved very healthy, in verbalizing his dislike of being told what to do.

The perspective changes somewhat as we think about how to present our expertise to adults. As part of interacting with our patients and clients on an adult-to-adult level, and in wanting to involve them in the therapy process, we ask the question, "What would you like to work on in therapy?" We expect that adults would want to be involved in decision making. When the client or family turns the question back with, "You tell me. You're the expert," we may be thrown off balance. That could, however, be a cue that they don't feel that they have enough information to make a good decision. What you described about the lawyer and the businessman seems to communicate not only the expectation that as therapists we behave as experts and take the responsibility for decisions, but also that we offer some guarantees. Patients and clients certainly have the right to know what they are purchasing as consumers of therapy (or medical) services, but we may need to help move them toward the idea of being an informed partner in the decision-making process. This may be an unfamiliar paradigm for their participation in health services but is one increasingly evident (Edmond, Pellagrino, Veatch, & Langan, 1991).

Part of the education we do with our patients and clients is to give them information so they can recognize their choices and make healthful decisions; at the same time, we as service providers must continue to be responsible and knowledgeable. When it comes to helping people to regain health and function optimally, we all know we can't make guarantees.

References

Cicchetti, D., Rogosch, F.A., & Toth, S.L. (1994). A developmental psychopathology perspective on depression in children and adolescents. In W.M. Reynolds & H.F. Johnston (Eds.), *Handbook of depression in children and adolescents*. New York: Plenum Press.

Edmond, D., Pellagrino, R.M., Veatch, R., & Langan, J.P. (Eds.). (1991). *Ethics, trust, and the professions: Philosophical and cultural aspects*. Washington, DC: Georgetown University Press.

Fine, S. (1990). Clinical case workbook II: Psychological issues and adaptive capacities. In C.B. Royeen (Ed.), *AOTA self-study series: Assessing function*. Rockville, MD: American Occupational Therapy Association.

Fine, S. (1993). Interaction between psychological variables and cognitive function. In C.B. Royeen (Ed.), *AOTA self-study series: Cognitive rehabilitation*. Rockville, MD: American Occupational Therapy Association.

CHAPTER 9

Community Context

KEY TOPICS

- Behavior modification
- Extinguishing behavior
- Traumatic brain injury
- Social skills training
- Modeling
- Cognitive strategies
- Community reentry
- Family's role and expectations

Initial Comments

As with our previous story, the following narrative focuses on a young man who has had a traumatic brain injury (TBI). In this instance, therapeutic intervention is overseen by a neuropsychologist who requests that all rehabilitation therapies coordinate their intervention through a behavioral program.

Behaviorism

The behaviorist tells us that as occupational therapists, we are behaviorists, for we are trying to change or enable people to change their behavior (Murdoch & Barker, 1991, p. 2). In its strictest sense, learning a behavior is demonstrated when specific information or stimuli in the environment evokes a new behavior. Simple behaviors combine to produce complex behaviors, or what we commonly refer to in occupational therapy as skills.

Learning theory or behaviorism has demonstrated that behaviors that are rewarded tend to be repeated, while those not followed by a desirable consequence tend to be abandoned or extinguished. What people find rewarding is related to how they get basic and secondary needs met. Rewards can be those we give ourselves (e.g., feelings of satisfaction or approval) or rewards that come from outside the self (e.g., money, praise, or attention). If you need approval, being praised will be rewarding to you. If you are tired, you might reward yourself for a hard day's work by settling down and putting your feet up. Reward is always related to need. All of this does not go on unconsciously; in fact, the individual is an active participant in the learning process. He or she becomes aware of personal needs and goals, and through personal experience (and by observing others) becomes aware of the consequences of behavior. Individuals learn to actively choose among competing rewards, to anticipate rewards, and to postpone action when needed. The ability to modulate one's response in this way depends on intact central nervous system function, and may be disrupted by TBI, as occurs in the following narrative.

Learning also involves the ability to discern the similarities among similar situations. Seeing these similarities allows people to generalize what they have learned in one setting to another. Likewise, people learn to discriminate among situations, noticing that situations are different and that the behaviors called for are different. The ability for generalization and discrimination is frequently disturbed by TBI.

Behavioral Assessment

In the behavioral practice model, the therapist is concerned with identifying what particular skills or behaviors contribute to adaptive function and skills that either are lacking or used ineffectively. Once desired skills are identified, the process of teaching skills can begin. Concurrently, the therapist looks to the milieu or treatment environment to see what in the environment either cues, supports, or detracts from building these desired skills.

Part of what detracts from optimum function may be the presence of undesirable or maladaptive behaviors. The therapist's assessment may include identifying what in the environment or activity reinforces or rewards maladaptive behavior. As discussed in the story of Nathan, the process of extinguishing undesirable behavior is that of judiciously eliminating rewards for this behavior. If a specific undesirable behavior is reinforced, even occasionally, rather than being extinguished, that behavior may become more firmly rooted.

Role of the Therapist in the Behavioral Model

Having identified the skills that need to be built or enhanced, the therapist must also identify current or potential rewards or reinforcers for behavior. When disease or disability drastically alters an individual's lifestyle, what had been rewarding may no longer be accessible or may no longer be experienced as rewarding. Basic needs—such as to give and receive love and approval, to feel satisfaction for what was accomplished, or the very basic need for nourishment and safety—do not change. The means by which these needs can be met and the criteria by which their achievement is measured can change dramatically.

The occupational therapist becomes somewhat of an environmental engineer, trying to ensure that desired behaviors are recognized and reinforced, and skills are learned and generalized to many situations. At the same time, the therapist tries to prevent undesirable behaviors from being rewarded, so they can be extinguished, and tries to help the person discriminate when specific behaviors are acceptable or unacceptable. New skills or behaviors must be taught to substitute for those eliminated; in other words, it's usually not enough to get people to stop meeting their needs in an inappropriate way—they need to learn an adaptive means to meet those needs.

The therapist also serves as a role model for appropriate social and task behavior, as we see in the story of Nathan. Given the behavioral emphasis of this story, please pay special attention to the feelings that seem to underlie the events described. Nathan is a young man who works hard to please his therapist while struggling to engage in his world, and in a manner in which he has integrity.

"Nathan" Narrated by Mary Ann Bruce, MS, OTR

Not long ago I treated an 18-year-old young man, Nathan, who had a TBI. His neuropsychologist called a team planning meeting to discuss a behavioral intervention plan designed to impact Nathan's social behavior. According to documentation, Nathan asked questions "constantly" and used about a dozen questions "repetitively" when relating to people at his home, in the community, or in the hospital. The kinds of questions he would ask included: "What's your favorite color?" "What's your favorite number?" "Where did you get...(usually an item of clothing)?" "What is your son's (daughter's, spouse's) name?" "What kind of work does your husband (wife) do?" and "What's your name?" The behavioral strategy suggested by the psychologist was ignoring or extinction.

Briefly, the psychologist requested that occupational therapy, speech therapy, and physical therapy do the following: (1) At the beginning of each therapy session, remind Nathan that his repetitive and excessive questions will be ignored. His questions are not to interrupt the therapy activity. (2) Restate the goal to him: ignoring his questions is to improve his "appropriate" interaction at home, in the community, and in therapy. (3) Reassure Nathan that we like him and are not being rude when we ignore his questions. (4) Each therapist is to identify a time when Nathan can ask (non–task-related) questions. The psychologist recommended the end of the treatment session. (5) Should Nathan ask questions not related to the current therapy task, therapists are to ignore him (no verbal or nonverbal response) and redirect him to the task in progress. The psychologist reminded us that when using extinction and ignoring strategies, the behavior may get worse before it gets better, but said we should see a change in behavior by the third session.

During this planning meeting, several specific situations and settings were identified by therapists and family members as situations where they believed change was desirable. These included Nathan's talking with everyone on the elevator; interrupting store clerks and hospital workers to ask for assistance or to "just be friendly"; distracting other clients during their outpatient therapy; asking store clerks and fast food servers their name, introducing himself, and shaking their hands; and behaviors directed toward getting the attention of mothers with small children (e.g., approaching mothers and asking their children's names).

As the occupational therapist who participated in community retraining (CRT) sessions weekly, I had observed or directly experienced most of these behavior situations and agreed that they posed a problem. I could understand his family's discomfort and embarrassment with some of Nathan's social behaviors, and I felt that these behaviors kept Nathan from establishing the kinds of social relationships that he desired.

Prior Strategies

Prior to this meeting, my strategy during my treatment sessions with Nathan had been to outline the session's task and review goals for physical, cognitive, and social function at the beginning of each CRT. I also outlined my expectation that there be no interruptions nor handshakes. If we were going into the community or were practicing such an outing, I reviewed the social expectations for a particular environment or posed questions to him in which he outlined the expected protocol. Initially, I had to verbally or nonverbally cue Nathan on how to behave in social settings while we were on our outings. I tried to avoid putting him in situations that would be too difficult for him to manage. I learned that when he was able to manage one environment (e.g., lunch at the hospital cafeteria), his ability for control and self-monitoring did not transfer to varied other settings (e.g., lunch at a burger stand). However, he did remember expectations for a particular environment when we returned to that same setting on several occasions. If left unattended, Nathan often initiated conversations with strangers, adults or children. I also noted that with fatigue (physical or mental), he required more frequent verbal cues and at times gave up, as he said, "trying to behave." At the end of each CRT session, we reviewed his accomplishments, and discussed the functional goals he achieved and the situations in which he met the challenge of better controlling his social behavior.

During each of these CRT wrap-up periods, he thanked me for helping him. I always reiterated that he had done the work: that I provided the framework for him. It was important to me that Nathan feel good about himself and give himself credit for all he had accomplished. However, one day as we were reviewing his accomplishments after an outing to a nearby mall, I felt as though his behavior was mostly to please me—I knew that he valued my opinions and approval. It seemed as though I had become an external motivator. My goal was for him to be internally motivated to change his social behavior, and to feel that he had some control and was doing things for himself.

I had tried many strategies in response to the personal questions he had posed to me. Initially, I responded to those questions about which I was comfortable sharing information. If he repeated questions, I reminded him that we had already discussed this and asked him to recall what I had said. Often, he initially wouldn't be able to recall, but after a couple of seconds he would remember and answer his own questions. Sometimes, I would answer his question and then ask him the same question. For example, if he asked, "How was your weekend?" I would answer, then ask about his. My goal was to recreate the kinds of everyday conversations people had.

I had also noticed that he repeated questions to get my attention; therefore, I sometimes responded by asking, "Would you like to talk about..." or "Let's talk about..." It struck me that he wanted to be social but did not know how to relate to the task at hand, nor how to initiate and maintain a conversation. He indicated that he liked to talk and wanted to learn to converse again. Previously, he had exceptional social skills and was seen as quite charming by adults and peers. Working on conversational skills in this way created a challenge to achieve occupational therapy goals and not step on the toes of the speech therapists who were working to develop his attention, cognitive abilities, and voice strength. They felt it was premature to address practical conversational skills.

He asked and frequently repeated some personal questions. I did not answer, and advised him that he should not ask personal questions (i.e., someone's age). Sometimes I answered his question and then we discussed when it was okay to pose such a query or we agreed upon other criteria that might form the boundaries for questions. Sometimes I felt he was being a typical adolescent in his communication style, but was unable to monitor its ineffectiveness when used with adults. For example, he frequently asked questions such as, "Where did you get those shoes?" or "Where did you get that ring?" I frequently hear adolescents talk about their belongings.

Before the team meeting to discuss the extinction program, a new speech therapist began to work with Nathan, and had tried a different behavior modification strategy. She had made five cards and on each card there was a question mark. These were used in a manner similar to tokens. Nathan was allowed to ask five questions during a 1-hour treatment period. For each question he asked the speech therapist, he had to give up a question card. Therefore, he had to evaluate if his question was important and whether or not he wanted to "spend" a card to ask it.

When his family described the program to me, they stated that the speech therapist wanted the other therapists, as well as family members, to use the strategy. I agreed, but was surprised by Nathan's response. He said he didn't want to do it and that it made him "feel stupid." Therefore, I did not force the issue and continued to use my other strategies.

Implementing the Extinction Program

The first time I tried to ignore his questions, I found it literally impossible. I was treating Nathan in his home, and he needed to use the restroom. While in the bathroom, he began to call my name. When I responded, assuming that he needed assistance, he asked me, "How much therapy time is left?" I gave him the time and then told him that I would talk to him when he was finished. I would be waiting for him in the kitchen. Within seconds, there was another call, and again he had a question not pertinent to the situation. I told him we would discuss it when he came out and please finish toileting and return to the kitchen. When therapy was over and I described the situation to his mother, she recounted similar experiences and the dilemma she and his father were in when they wanted to ignore him but were afraid he needed assistance. However, they had come up with a good response in asking, "Is it an emergency?" They were helping him learn that only in an emergency should he do his talking from the bathroom. She also said she felt embarrassed when he did this while his friends were visiting.

Given this experience in his home, I began to anticipate what strategies I could use to ignore behavior and questions in the community. I wondered if it was realistic to ignore his questions in the community. I was aware of two issues: (1) my own lack of comfort with the program and (2) the reality of situations outside of clinical environments. After considering both of these issues, I decided to combine several strategies on our next CRT—a trip to the library.

Before entering the library, I sat down on a bench to review the treatment plan with Nathan. As usual, I asked him what he perceived as the goal for today's CRT. His response was "Get a book," and he got up to walk inside. I asked him to sit down and stated that I wanted to review the new program that Dr. I.C. wanted us to try. He then added, "I'm not supposed to ask inappropriate questions." I asked him if he understood the reasons for that and what he believed would be inappropriate for this experience (using the library). He said his parents didn't want him to ask questions and he didn't know what would be inappropriate for this setting. I then spent a few moments helping him identify a benefit for himself, not just his parents. We focused on the self-image that he wanted to have—that of an adult. We then identified what appropriate questions he might use. For instance, he might ask for help to find a book or ask for instructions for doing a computer search. We also discussed things he should avoid (e.g., interrupting people reading, doing their job, or browsing in the library). I also asked him to tell me how long he wanted to be in the library before he took a break. He set the goal of 30 minutes doing his search and using questions as needed. Nathan successfully met his goal of asking limited and appropriate questions for 30 minutes and requested directions for finding the bathroom when he needed to use the facility. After 30 minutes, we went outside for a break. I gave him positive feedback and we agreed to go back inside and find the book we had identified on the computer search.

Discussion Questions

1. What have you learned from this story?
2. Have you ever been involved in implementing or have you observed a behavior modification program such as the one suggested by the neuropsychologist in this story?
   a. In what ways was it similar or unlike the behavior approach recommended for Nathan?
   b. What enhanced or seemed to stand in the way of positive outcomes with the behavioral programs you have witnessed?
3. Identify the feelings conveyed by Nathan in this story.
   a. How are these addressed by staff?
   b. Do you feel that they are adequately addressed? What is the basis for your opinion?
4. Discuss the feelings expressed by Nathan's parents.
   a. Have you in your personal life or professional role known parents whose children have had impairing disorders? What do these parents struggle with?
   b. How can occupational therapists help these families deal with emotional issues?
5. The neuropsychologist recommends a behavioral program that minimizes cognitive demands, while the narrating therapist describes having previously incorporated many cognitive strategies. Compare the two approaches in terms of what is expected of the patient and the potential benefits to the patient.
6. The therapist also tries to model communication and social behavior. Review your information on modeling theory and contrast the therapist's approach with the theoretical recommendations.
   a. What attributes of the occupational therapist increase the likelihood that Nathan will try to model her behavior?
   b. What attributes decrease this likelihood?
7. If you had been the occupational therapist treating this patient, what behavioral strategies might you have tried, and based on what behavioral assumptions?
8. What are some community activities that can be used with young adults with chronic mental disorders or long-term cognitive impairments toward the goal of community reintegration?
9. Discuss how you would structure social skills training for Nathan (e.g., How could you build practical skills related to increasing patience? Learning to ask questions appropriately?).
10. What factors need to be considered when implementing a behavior modification program? Give examples from this narrative that illustrate these (e.g., therapist's comfort, safety concerns, client concerns).

Impressions

MAB: The neuropsychologist and speech therapist in this example are recommending classic behavior modification approaches. As the occupational therapist, I was incorporating cognitive behavioral strategies. Rather than ignoring the client's inappropriate questions in order to extinguish them, I'm giving him information designed to help him assess, on the spot, when and if particular questions are appropriate. I also was using modeling. The issue for me is, are these various strategies compatible in this instance, or are they working at odds with each other?

I think this story highlights the difficulty of implementing a behavioral program in the community. We usually can't take the risk of ignoring questions or requests for assistance when we're not certain if the client is safe, for instance, and we often need to intervene if he or she is disturbing people in public places. Also, stores, restaurants, and malls are much more stimulating than the familiar arena of the clinic setting. There are many more variables to contend with.

The treatment staff in this story emphasized to the patient that they didn't ignore his questions because of a dislike for him. I've worked with several clients who appeared to have trouble understanding this, and would more often see staff who ignored them as disliking or being unconcerned about them, or even punishing them.

Clients also may misinterpret the intent of family members who implement behavior modification programs at home. I recall a young woman with a brain injury who felt her mother hated her and was punishing her. Family members can become fatigued with implementing the program, which usually is a long-term process for people with severe brain injury. The mother, here the primary caregiver, stressed by the slow progress of the program, became irritable and could not effectively implement the program. The result was a mother-daughter relationship characterized by tension and impatience, hostility and anger, and little effective communication and cooperation by mother or daughter. For me, this example emphasizes the importance of close monitoring and ongoing reevaluation of these programs.

When behavior modification programs are used with young adults, they may need adaptation to accommodate other needs. I know there is literature supporting behavior modification programs for managing behavior problems that result from TBI. However, in the previous story and related example, both clients are young adults, and I feel that in spite of their injuries, both clients have adult developmental needs for control and independence which conflict with the behavioral control strategies.

BB: If Nathan can improve his social skills, he's going to be better able to connect with other people as he needs and desires. When I began reading this story, I worried that Nathan, the person, was going to get lost in the behavioral program. As the story unfolds, I get more a sense of the person-to-person relationship between you and Nathan.

As described, the behavior plan proposed by the psychologist doesn't appear to be one that would extinguish the behavior of asking non–task-related questions; rather, its design supports having non–task-related questions postponed until therapeutic activities have been completed. It's not a program for extinction but one that tries to increase discrimination learning. During his therapy sessions, Nathan has to make an important discrimination. Is this a therapy session in progress? If so, questions are to pertain only to the task. Is the therapeutic task complete? Then other questions are permissible. A second discrimination may be much more complicated. He has to assess, "Is the question I'm asking related to the therapy task?" I'm not certain that we know from the story if he consistently can make that determination. Also, I didn't gather that the nature of acceptable post-session questions had been specified. As the occupational therapist, you were working to teach Nathan how to incorporate casual (non–task-related) questions and dialogue into a more natural flow within the therapy session. And, as you indicated, you were trying to increase Nathan's ability for discrimination through your use of cues within your dialogue with him. (I refer the reader to Chapter 12 for additional information about cognitive intervention.) It's apparent that one of your concerns was that behaviors not be eliminated without something being learned in their place. I think your comment about Nathan being like other adolescents and young adults in wanting to talk about clothes or possessions helps remind us that his having brain impairment doesn't keep him from being what he is—a young adult. This young man wants to have tools that will enable him to have casual conversations just like other 18-year-olds.

Outings seem complicated if you're being highly behavioral. How does a therapist control the responses of others to Nathan's overtures during an outing in the community? For instance, if he approaches a mother in the supermarket to ask about her children, I'd imagine some women would be put off, but others would be eager to respond. Therapists can ignore inappropriate questions, but these questions aren't as likely to be ignored by others in the community—even if they get negative attention. I'm aware that one strategy has been to videotape these kinds of encounters in the community so clients take a careful look at their own behavior and the reaction of others to their behavior. That, too, helps their discrimination learning.

I thought an important lesson in this story was in the comments you made about using strategies that would enhance Nathan's ability for self-control. For example, since appropriate social behavior required a great deal of concentration and energy, you helped Nathan take breaks so he could reconstitute. That's going to help his self-confidence. It's worth reminding ourselves that in this instance, mental effort can be just as fatiguing as physical.

In both this story and the one before, I tried to imagine what the families of these two young men might have been going through. The mother in this story mentions feeling embarrassed. I'm sure that doesn't begin to capture the grief, loss, frustration, and worry that she and Nathan's father must experience, probably over and over again, as they see their son so changed. As parents, we have hopes for our children, not necessarily for great things, but for a healthy and fulfilling life. For these families, the future's uncertainty must seem daunting, rather than full of promise.

References

Murdoch, D., & Barker, P. (1991). *Basic behaviour therapy.* Oxford: Blackwell Scientific Publications.

CHAPTER 10

Personal Meaning of Objects

KEY TOPICS

- Objects and their meaning
- Depression
- Grief
- Lost and misplaced belongings
- Role of family in treatment
- Behavior modification
- Behavioral frame of reference
- Disengagement
- Role of occupational therapy with terminally ill clients

An artist tells the following story:

"I was in my gallery one day when a woman came in and asked if I had any calendars illustrated with my work. She wanted to purchase a gift for a friend who was terminally ill. This customer said that her friend had 2 or 3 months to live. The woman in the gallery hoped that in buying her friend a calendar, she would communicate the message that this friend had to live out the calendar year. We got to talking and I felt myself becoming involved with these two women's stories. Before she left, I gave the woman a piece of bear fur that I had cut from a bear hide that had been given to me. I asked her to give it to her ill friend. I saw bears as a symbol of strength as well as of death and rebirth, and I wanted to share that.

"About a year and a half later, I was in my gallery and a woman who I had never met came up to me and asked if I was...(name of artist). When I said 'Yes,' she responded by introducing herself, and added, 'You saved my life.'

"She went on to say that 2 years before she had been very ill and had been told by all of her doctors that she had only a short time to live. There was a surgical procedure these physicians wanted to try, but they gave her little hope that it would be successful. The woman said that a friend of hers had given her a calendar and a piece of bear fur. This woman stated, 'I knew I was very sick and I felt that all my thoughts had been focused on my illness. So, I decided to try and clear my thoughts and focus on this piece of bear hide. I put it in a small pouch which I hung around my neck. For some time each day, I tried to clear my mind of all other thoughts and just visualize the bear fur. I had surgery and lived through it, which wasn't expected. And there were more surgeries to follow. In each instance, before my surgery, I was told I would have to remove the pouch hanging around my neck because it wasn't sterile. But I was starting to believe that this pouch and its contents were important to me and I refused to remove them. I told the nurses and doctors, "If I'm as sick as you say, what difference can an unsterile pouch around my neck make?" They let me keep it on. It's been over a year now, and I've been pronounced healthy. When I go see my physicians, I pat my rosy cheeks and say to them, "Looking pretty good for someone who's not supposed to be alive, aren't I?"'"

The artist continues:

"The woman who was telling me this story said she felt that in having to fight to hold on to her pouch and the snippet of fur inside she was fighting back against the medical people who had told her she wouldn't live, and that she also was fighting against her illness. For me it was a powerful story that had meaning on many levels."

Initial Comments

By their very nature, stories are meant to be shared, and we begin this chapter with a story that was told to us. If we try to identify just what the piece of bear hide "meant" or how the process of taking care of it was healing, we'd be liable to distract from rather than add to what is within the story itself. Yet this account provides a vivid example of the potential significance of personal objects and their place within meaningful occupation.

The Significance of Personal Objects

We know that personal belongings take on meaning in our lives. We often dispose of belongings that don't have meaning. For our purposes, we refer to those tangible but nonhuman objects we obtain in life or that we gather around us through the course of our lives. Virtually every theoretical framework we can identify in occupational therapy, psychology or psychiatry, sociology, and anthropology can tell us something about the role of objects in the human experience, although from slightly different vantages. We know, for instance, that objects can range from "necessary tools or implements to frivolous adornments" (Kielhofner, 1985, p. 45). Objects are part of our rituals; they are a part of work, play, and daily routines. Like a teddy bear, they can bring us comfort; like a weapon, they can hurt us or be a means of fighting back. We acquire objects to identify who we are, our interests, and our status. We wear them to show that we are like or separate from our peers. We remember people and special times by the gifts we give or are given and the souvenirs we buy. Through objects, we can demonstrate our love or benevolence or try to make up for indiscretions. We don't have to do anything with our objects, but may simply place them around our environment. Some objects can be easily replaced by others; for instance, if I can't have that Ford, I'll have this Ford, or that Chevy; other objects are irreplaceable. Some objects we create with our own hands; others represent the technological culture we live in. Objects become associated with times in our lives and periods in our development: that treadmill that represented our determination to become healthier may be put aside for the books that signify our newer interest in a college degree; the pillbox with its little compartments and the lifeline on the bedside stand attest to a period of medical struggles. At times we gather objects, and at times and with great intention, we may leave them behind. Giving objects away can be very freeing when objects have become an encumbrance, or are too much or too many to care for. We know, too, that losing an object can make us grieve, for objects can become very special and their loss brings sadness. If each of us were to tell the story of our lives, we could do so by letting the objects we sought, cherished, lost, neglected, or mourned speak for us.

Introduction to "The Dress"

The stories in this chapter place a spotlight on objects that are significant in the lives of the main figures. These narratives share also an underlying theme of loss, a theme especially striking in the first story entitled "The Dress." It is the story of an older woman who has experienced several losses and now grieves. In a way, the object lost seems to represent many other losses.

Grief as a Response to Loss

Grief involves intense feelings of emotional suffering, and is a normal response to loss (Burnell & Burnell, 1989). It is not identical to the clinical syndromes of depression (e.g., major depression or dysthymia), although feelings of sadness and a depressed affect are parts of the grief process. Both grief and depression may include physical/motor changes, withdrawal from activities formerly enjoyed, and cognitive changes, including preoccupation. Grief is a part of the healing process, and the grieving individual must accept loss as painful and accept the changes that loss brings (Burnell & Burnell, 1989).

Occupational therapists frequently work with individuals who have had or are experiencing a variety of losses. Physical and psychological conditions often bring about life changes and subsequent losses around one's expected length and quality of life. While not an exhaustive list, losses can include those related to roles and abilities, significant relationships, status and wage-earning, independence, and sense of physical and emotional well-being.

When, as occupational therapists, we are around persons who are grieving, we have an excellent opportunity to practice active listening and provide support. If we are to help people work through the grief process, we need to be comfortable with our own feelings, and tolerate the feelings of sadness, even despair, that may be communicated as part of the grieving process. This is illustrated in the following story.

"The Dress" (Anonymous)

Recently, I was the per diem therapist employed for the day on a transitional care unit. In preparation for the day's work, I was given guides for treatment for each patient assigned. Mrs. N., who was 80 years old, was recovering from a hip fracture. I was to help her with her ADLs.

After I had helped her finish her personal care, she told me that the one dress she owned and wished to wear was in the closet. I went over to the closet to get her dress, but found that the closet was empty. When I told her that her dress wasn't there, to my surprise she began to cry hysterically. "That's my only dress...I have nothing to wear...Someone stole my beautiful dress with pink roses. What can I do?...When they brought me here they didn't even care...the lady just took it off and threw it in the laundry bag."

Although I tried to calm her, I was unable to comfort her nor could I stop her crying. After about 10 minutes of listening and reassuring her that I would help her find something to wear, hopefully her favored dress, she began to sob quietly.

First I made certain that she was safe in her wheelchair and clothed in a clean hospital gown. Then I went to the laundry room to ask about her dress. I was told to check the clean clothes rack and I did so, but my efforts were in vain. Before I had to give the bad news to Mrs. N., I inquired if there were other places to look for lost clothing. Nursing staff suggested I speak to the social worker. After waiting 10 minutes to see a very busy social worker, I was told to go to the laundry room. After hearing that I had done this, she told me where I could borrow clothes for this patient to use until hers could be found.

Regretting that I had to tell Mrs. N. that I was unable to find her favorite dress, I entered her room to find that she was sitting where I had left her but was now calm. When I told her that I could not locate her dress and presented her with the loaner dress, she began to sob again. But what she talked about changed. She began to describe the recent death of her husband and how she had cared for him. She discussed fears about having no one to take care of her, and questioned aloud how she could take care of herself since she had broken her hip.

Although I would have liked to have spent more time with her, I had other patients waiting. I helped her dress and listened to her concerns for a bit longer, and supported her as best I could. Then I excused myself and told her that she would have an opportunity to problem solve with the social worker. I added that I would leave a note for the social worker and the nurse so they could continue to give her support in this very difficult time.

Discussion Questions

1. What feelings did this story stir in you?
2. What would your response to this individual have been had you been the therapist?

3. Therapists frequently hear residents describe the loss of personal belongings. Residents sometimes suggest that the items were stolen either by staff or by other residents or patients. They also are discouraged by the frequency in which items are misplaced by nursing staff or lost or ruined in the laundry. As the occupational therapist, how would you respond to a patient or resident who insisted a personal item had been stolen by another client or a staff member?
4. Have you ever lost an especially important object or personal belonging, or had one taken from you?
   a. Describe what that was like for you.
   b. Why do suppose the loss was so significant at the time?
5. Develop a system (laundry, organizing, or accounting for personal belongings) that could prevent some of the problems exemplified in this story.
6. Are there specific occupational therapy activities that you might use in groups to help clients cope with loss? Identify activities you could use with younger as well as middle-aged and older clients.

Impressions

BB: This story reminds me of others I've heard, including in my own family. I've seen patients and clients get really angry when their possessions are lost; some express disgust, and others, as in this story, become very sad. There are people who have never taken off their wedding ring or a special necklace, who are told they must remove them because of concerns about safety or infection, and then they never get them back. It can be tremendously unsettling. I wonder if in some of these instances there aren't several things going on. One is the loss itself added to the many other losses that may be occurring. Another is the (now violated) trust that, "If you (medical people) can take care of my things, I can count on you to take care of me." I know of one woman who had her dress misplaced at a general hospital. When it was time for her to go home, the staff brought someone else's clothes. The lady said, "But these aren't mine!" The staff member responded first with, "Are you sure?" as if the patient didn't have all her mental faculties. And then the staff person suggested, "Well, why don't you wear these anyway?" We can only imagine the interesting chain of events this set off. Fortunately, a nurse heard her protests, found the missing clothes, and set things straight.

We can't know what this dress signifies for the woman in this story, but clearly she had much she needed to grieve. Sometimes patients or clients lose or misplace their own things, and they mistakenly blame others, but I doubt that diminishes the feelings of loss they experience at the time.

MAB: This scenario draws attention to multiple issues around loss: the loss of personal belongings, the loss of a spouse, the loss of ability to care for oneself, and the significance of the loss of personal and material resources. I would have a hard time deciding which of these is the worst or most painful. I guess each person has different values that affect his or her reaction to loss. However, of all the losses I see, it seems that the strongest feeling of burden occurs when a person can no longer care for himself or herself. Throughout life, we grieve as we give up familiar places, people, and objects. Over time, we live with this sadness, and somehow it becomes tolerable. But when we lose the ability to be independent in self-care, it not only brings about a sense of loss and sadness, but seems to have a multidimensional impact on our quality of life—and usually gets worse rather than better, especially for the older adult, or people with severe or multiple disabilities. I remember a young man with poor balance and motor control who was unable to clean himself after a bowel movement and had to have his mother assist him with hygiene. I'll never forget the gratitude he expressed when I was able to structure his environment so he could give up diapers, shave himself, and achieve independence in self-care with the proper setup. He said to me, "Thank you—you've made me feel normal." His function was still not "normal," but his words and the look on his face expressed a depth of feeling about what being independent in self-care meant. I can't find the words to describe adequately the impact of this client's statement.

Introduction to "Objects d'Art"

The next story takes place in a client's home. The main individual seems no longer to have interest in her therapy, nor in other areas of her daily life. The referral to occupational therapy is to help motivate this woman to reengage. The story illustrates the integral place that objects have in this individual's life, and overall, it serves as an example of using activity to achieve a therapeutic goal.

Significance of Depression

Interestingly, the word "depression" never appears in this story, but one can wonder to what extent the woman in the next story may be experiencing a significant depression. Some of the classical signs of depression include lack of interest and pleasure in activity, withdrawal from former activities, minimal motivation, hopelessness, tearfulness, and sleep and eating disturbances. In his discussion of depression, Wenar (1994) identifies depression as emanating from two kinds of loss: the loss of a significant other or the loss of self-worth (pp. 189-190). Many of our clients are faced with both kinds of loss. While the client described in the story seems to manifest several signs of depression and has motivational problems, we know, too, that motivation and depression can be influenced by a variety of other factors that could be significant for this woman, including the use of medication and central nervous system disturbances related to her cerebral vascular accident. For her, the decision has been to take a behavioral approach to treatment.

Individualizing Treatment in the Behavioral Model

If, as in this story, one is assessing the possibility of using behavioral techniques to modify a patient's or client's behavior, there are questions to be asked which will enable the therapist to individualize therapy to meet the particular values, concerns, abilities, and limitations of each particular client. In this story, these questions might include,

"What does this woman need to achieve through her behavior?" "What does she enjoy or find rewarding?" "What behaviors can she be reasonably expected to achieve?" and "How can one be certain that the goals and behaviors identified for treatment are those that she desires?" Given this chapter's focus on the meaningfulness of objects, we'd like you to think also about what role objects in the milieu, here books and decorative objects, have in this woman's life.

"Objects d'Art" Narrated by Mary Ann Bruce, MS, OTR

While working for a home health agency, I was asked to reevaluate a woman who had had a massive basilar stroke approximately 1 year earlier. The referral was for assessment only. The purpose of the evaluation was to identify additional daily living activities that the client could relearn and to determine how occupational therapy could work with the psychologist who was establishing a behavior modification program in response to her decreased motivation for and cooperation with treatment. Presenting problems included severe upper extremity ataxia, poor sitting and standing balance, an attention span of approximately 10 minutes, and dependency for self-care (feeding, grooming, bathing, personal hygiene, and dressing). A significant problem, too, was that the woman seemed to be losing her motivation to use the abilities she had. Because she was limited in her verbal communication ability, her family members (her husband and a college-aged daughter) provided information about her medical history, the course of rehabilitation, her current daily routine, and previous lifestyle.

The woman, who was in her late 40s, had been a prominent lawyer in the community, had an active family and social life, and pursued her interest in the arts through volunteer activities when her other roles allowed. Her interest in the arts was reflected throughout her home, beginning with the beautifully landscaped gardens and moving to the meticulously designed interior and the original Southwestern art displayed throughout her home.

As the evaluation progressed, the family's caring attitude and interest in contributing to a quality of life for the client was evident. They had pursued training in nonmedical alternative therapies, as well as learning exercises they could help her with on the Swiss ball. Six months previously, therapies had been discontinued because the client had failed to progress. That was when the family had established a home therapy routine which they were still implementing. During that period, the client had been cooperative, but recently she appeared to have lost interest and was becoming increasingly resistive to any therapy experience. The family asked for ideas to increase her participation and verbalized that they were willing to try a behavior modification program which her neuropsychologist had recommended, but not without reservation. He had recommended that the client's reward for participating in her daily therapy would be that she go out with her daughter when she walked the dog. The family described the client's previous interests as her dog, gardening, reading, her job, and art. Given the pleasure the client received from being with her dog and being outside in the beautiful community, they were uncomfortable withholding these outings from her should she fail to meet her therapy goals. Therefore, they asked if I had any other ideas for promoting the client's cooperation and participation in their home therapy program.

Before making any suggestions, I asked them to show me the exercise routine and explain the daily program. I also asked to see her eat to evaluate the concerns they expressed about her upper extremity ataxia. When I watched the client eat, I saw that she could manage finger foods but could not safely use utensils. The family was aware of her limitations, but hoped to help her learn to use a utensil. They felt this might motivate her to eat. She had apparently lost interest in food, and no longer ate the foods she had enjoyed previously. Often, the family fed her to assure that she had adequate nutrition. I wondered if both the client and her family might be uncomfortable with the childish image of her eating food with her fingers.

Her husband had built an area to serve as an adapted standing table, and it was quite innovative. However, the client now refused to stand. As I evaluated the situation and listened to their comments, it seemed that she lacked a reason to stand at a table. In itself, standing at a table was not very satisfying. I began to look around the room for ideas. I noticed several bookcases, one with cookbooks and various other subjects and a second one filled with books depicting the work of renowned artists. Again I looked around to see paintings, sculpture, and tapestry throughout her home. Although I am not sure if it was my own desire to enjoy the art in these books or an occupational therapy motive, I suggested that we test her standing endurance while we browsed through one of her favorite books. Occasionally, she would look up at one of the paintings or sculptures within our view. The client maintained attention for about 15 minutes without signs of fatigue. I am not sure if it was the novelty or the opportunity to pursue an interest and enjoy meaningful objects that supported her involvement. Because she could not verbalize her thoughts, I never will know. I recommended that the family continue to try to direct her attention to an activity of interest while simultaneously working toward the goal of increased standing tolerance.

Discussion Questions

1. Discuss the role of meaningful objects in occupational therapy evaluation and treatment. How can the therapist elicit information about objects of interest?
2. Assume that you were the occupational therapist. What other intervention strategies could you try that use this client's interests to promote her participation in therapy?
3. Discuss your view of the behavior modification program suggested by the neuropsychologist to promote participation by the client in her home therapy program.
4. When adults lose their ability to meet previous performance standards, they may become embarrassed and frequently lose interest in therapy tasks or previous activities pursued at home, work, or in the community. What physical, cognitive, and psy-

chosocial factors may be contributing to this client's loss of interest in eating and her decreased participation in her daily therapy program implemented by the family?

5. What role do you see the family taking in this client's therapy?
6. Does it seem that the family has realistic expectations for the client? What factors would you consider to evaluate their expectations for function?
7. If this woman wants to discontinue therapy, what ethical principles would guide your behavior as her therapist? What if, as may be the case, you cannot establish for certain what her desires are?
8. How might you articulate to a family your assessment that their loved one is not likely to profit further from therapy?

Impressions

MAB: Recalling this experience reminds me of the conflict that this family and others experience. Families struggle with balancing hope for the client's future with realistic expectations. This family seems committed to the patient's quality of life and hopes that she will be able to achieve a higher level of function. I didn't know whether or not this woman would be able to achieve more in the future. It's often difficult for therapists and families to know when it's time to consider that there may not be further improvement.

When considering this woman's decreased interest in food, I believe that this was an indication of her depression as much as of her inability to use utensils. I feel that many times in therapy when patients are uncooperative or seem to have a change in their level of interest, it relates to depression. When you're depressed, the tasks involved in therapy seem to take energy you no longer have. Since this woman cannot speak coherently, it becomes more complicated to assess the extent of her depression.

BB: Given your description of this woman, she has experienced tremendous loss and could understandably become depressed. There also is the stress and fatigue of trying to control her body in space. For her, just staying upright is a battle. We don't have enough information to know how she might be dealing with her feelings, nor do we know what she perceives as the likelihood that she can improve. Maybe she has begun to believe that she's not going to improve. This woman communicates something very important through her resistance, but we aren't sure what it is. Is she expressing discouragement? Has she given up, or does she want a time out from the demands of therapy? Does she dislike the therapeutic activities? Are her resistance to therapy and reluctance to eat related to depression? Or is she trying to find a way to take some control in her life? As much as her family wants the best for her, they don't necessarily know what she wants for herself. I would like to know more about how this woman communicates, then do everything I could to try to understand what she is communicating. It seems that you, the therapist, have engaged the client in an activity that she finds meaningful and motivating. Beyond that, it seems that you both have communicated through your mutual enjoyment of art, and that may prove just as important.

As therapists, we see people every day that exhibit a will to go on and struggle against great odds. Surely it becomes overwhelming at times, and people get worn down. We began our text with stories about the need individuals have to exert control. I often have felt that when people are depressed, it relates in part to their perception that they have no control over the events of their lives, that nothing they do is going to "matter" anyway. I would be very cautious about using a program, behavioral or other, that would in any way take control from this woman. But having said that, I know, too, that sometimes there are impasses in therapy—moments when nothing seems to be happening. If we can help our clients get past these, they sometimes thank us later on for helping them to keep going. The issues in this story are complex, and for me, relate to how best to keep the client at-center, to give her information that she can understand, and to ensure that her wishes are respected.

Introduction to "Leah"

In contrast to the clients who had meaningful objects that they wanted to keep or enjoy, the client in this story describes getting rid of all of her belongings and moving into the "nursing home" to await death from cancer. The narrating therapist comments that, in her view, this woman is grieving. Notice how grief is expressed differently in this story than it was in the two preceding accounts.

As with several of our other stories, there are subtle but significant instances in which the therapist gives the client as much control as possible during their interaction. The narrator also describes being asked to share personal information. Students frequently ask, "How much about myself should I share with my patients?" and there is no right answer. While personal sharing seems comfortable and supportive for the client in this story, in other instances it may prove confusing or problematic. Self-disclosure depends partly on the client's ability to be boundaried and to use the information appropriately, and on the therapist's own comfort and degree to which he or she wishes to share.

"Leah" Narrated by Mary Ann Bruce, MS, OTR

One Saturday morning, while providing occupational therapy weekend coverage, I had the pleasure of working with Leah, a patient in a skilled nursing facility. She was on my schedule with a note from her primary therapist advising me not to be intimidated by Leah's sarcastic sense of humor and to be sensitive to her constant pain. Leah had an inoperable brain mass. I was to assist her as needed to groom and dress at bedside and help as needed for bed mobility and safe wheelchair transfer.

When I entered Leah's room, which she shared with two other women, she informed me that she was having a "tough day" but indicated that she wanted to freshen up and get dressed. She made sarcastic remarks about occupational therapy but seemed relieved that I didn't go away. I still haven't figured out what she was communicating by her sarcasm. Sometimes, I felt as though it was a test of my trustworthiness; other times, I felt that it was her way of managing her feelings of anger and expressing humor.

During the 75 minutes in which we worked, she expressed pleasure in the feel of a warm cloth on her face. She seemed embarrassed that I had to help her wash her back, but was relieved that she was able to wash her own "peri" area. She apologized for having to rest after each bedside bathing task.

As I helped her dress, she said that she had just gotten rid of all of her personal belongings. She proceeded to describe how she had sold her home and most of her personal belongings to cover the costs of her care during her "last days" in the "nursing home." Some things, however, she had given away. She stated that she no longer needed much anyway. When she was dressed, I asked if she was ready to transfer to her wheelchair and be up for a while. She indicated that she was quite fatigued and would prefer to stay in bed a bit longer. I abided by her request and said I would return later to help her up and finish her therapy program. In the meantime, I would assist other patients with their morning routines.

About 2 hours later when I returned to her room she had just returned from her physical therapy session and was fatigued. However, she said, "I am never too tired to talk. Tell me about yourself." I told her I could stay a few minutes and we could get to know each other. I briefly shared some information about my family and told her I was a student. I then inquired about her life history. She described a 40-year marriage with a loving spouse who was deceased about 3 years. She spoke of their decision not to have children, and she talked about some of her interests and career experiences.

Needless to say, this took longer than a few minutes, but at the end of our talk she stated that she would like to get up and go to occupational therapy. During the discussion, she commented that she was relieved that she could still read but frustrated by her hand tremors. Although she could still perform fine motor tasks, she was displeased with the quality of work she could produce and the increased time required to perform tasks. When we arrived at the clinic I suggested that she practice writing her name. She enthusiastically agreed and said she wanted to send thank you notes for all of the flowers she had received from friends while in the hospital recently. While she took a break from working on her penmanship, she described more of her life experiences and talked about her home and garden.

I sensed that she was grieving the loss of her home and adjusting to the idea of ending her life in a nursing home. She seemed relieved that she no longer had to care for her possessions. It was interesting to hear her describe how she had given her things to friends who would enjoy or care for them. The objects that she had chosen to keep and bring with her to the nursing facility were books, a few clothes, and a radio. After hearing about her previous interest in drawing and painting, I suggested that she ask a friend to bring her some drawing pencils, pastels, or watercolors. I told her we could help her use these in therapy.

Several weeks passed. Leah graduated from occupational therapy and proudly displayed her certificate of accomplishment in her room. Although she was no longer my patient, each Saturday I took a few minutes to run in and say hello to her.

For several weeks, Leah avoided asking a friend for her paints, and I never asked why. Then one week she told me she had her paints and had begun to paint the tree outside her window. She showed me her initial efforts. She seemed pleased with what she had painted. On two occasions during the weeks that followed, I asked about her painting. The first time she simply said, "I haven't gotten back to that yet." The next time she informed me that she wasn't driven to finish it and that she only painted when she felt like it and if it was pleasurable. That reminded me of the importance of pleasure compared to productivity.

Each week when I visit she seems glad to see me and lately has told me about a book she is reading. Two weeks ago, she told me that her doctor said her extensive chemotherapy was effective and her cancer is in remission. She followed this good news with her view that "...perhaps giving up all my responsibilities and the pressure of caring for things has helped me...it's good I'm here. It's helping me." Since hearing this news, I have noticed that she is paying more attention to her appearance and is initiating interaction with her roommate. I don't sense that she regrets selling or giving away her belongings, but I do sense that she may need more stimulation than this environment currently provides.

Discussion Questions

1. What did you learn from this story?
2. Compare the grief response in this story to the one in the "The Dress."
3. Have you ever worked with people who have life-threatening illness? How was that experience for you?
4. Discuss what you see as the role of occupational therapy in intervention with persons having life-threatening illness.
    a. Given the client's prognosis, what criteria might be used to determine the appropriateness of occupational therapy service?
5. What is the role of the client's meaningful objects as described in this story?
6. If you were in similar circumstances as this patient, what objects would you choose to have with you in this setting?
7. Discuss how you have seen humor, including sarcasm, ease difficult therapy situations. Has it ever seemed destructive? If so, in what way?

Impressions

BB: This story may seem to have two installments because it was written in two parts, the second portion of which begins with the words, "Several weeks passed." The first portion seems to be about disengaging, the second about reengaging. The image I'm most drawn to is that of the tree that Leah chooses to depict, an image that beautifully represents the story's shift.

In our stories, we have not addressed the use of humor as a means of coping. In this story, the therapist comments about Leah's sarcasm, which sounds like it was both hostile and humorous. I've encountered that often with my own clients. It's something I try to roll with rather then become defensive about. In fact, clients often make it easier for both of us to deal with difficult procedures or topics when they introduce humor. It allows us to acknowledge, though not in so many words, that this is a tough issue or a hard day. We know that sometimes sarcasm is a person's indirect way of letting us know that he or she is upset with us. If I sense that, I try to help the individual be more direct; first, by letting the client know that he or she sounds upset, then, by asking if there's something I have done or something going on that he or she would like to talk about.

I was glad to read your comment in the story about the importance of doing activities for the pleasure they bring, and not just for their outcome. I think we tend to be more tuned in to that when we work with children than with adults.

MAB: This story reminds me of other instances in which the loss or acquisition of objects became very important in people's lives. I've worked with a number of younger and middle-aged persons who were terminally ill and making decisions regarding their possessions and their careers, and arranging for the care of their loved ones. Their decisions demonstrated the personal meaning of objects, the relationship of objects to interests, and the role of objects in the varied process of disengagement. And, although their object choices might change, clients often continue to need the stimulation that objects can bring, and they often want to maintain their relationship with certain possessions associated with pleasure, strength, skills, or independence.

I recall one young man, a successful architect, who described his sorrow at not being able to drive due to frequent seizures, and the need to sell his red sports car. What he talked about was not just a vehicle but a longtime friend that brought him pleasure, provided transportation and independence, and fit his image. When he talked about selling his car, he grieved the loss of a successful image. He went on to describe selling his business and the frustration and sadness he felt from giving up familiar objects and longtime interests, and his fear of financial insecurity.

Not only do patients give up objects, new ones also may come into their lives as they become increasingly disabled. For example, this same architect now stumbled and frequently fell, and could no longer go for his daily run. He hated and refused to use his AFO to improve his gait and was convinced that exercise would strengthen his legs for safe walking. Until then, he said he would hold on to his wife's arm when he was out in the community. At home, he stabilized himself by holding on to furniture. Although he described a history of falls, he was unable to believe or accept therapists' recommendations that he use his AFO and a walker. Unlike Leah, he was not ready to let go of life. In terms of his age, he was in the prime period for adult achievement but now was unable to be as productive as he wished. This in turn influenced his feelings about objects and their significance in his life.

References

Burnell, G., & Burnell, A. (1989). *Clinical management of bereavement.* New York: Human Sciences Press.

Kielhofner, G. (1985). *A model of human occupation.* Baltimore: Williams and Wilkins.

Wenar, C. (1994) *Developmental psychology: From infancy through adolescence.* New York: McGraw-Hill.

CHAPTER 11

Reengagement

KEY TOPICS

- Occupational therapy outreach to homeless persons
- Community reentry
- Older adult
- Responding to withdrawn individual
- Grief
- Symbolic communication
- The arts in occupational therapy

Initial Comments

It can be very difficult to put into words how or why certain events and activities take on a special significance. At one level, and without wishing to use terms lightly, we could say that at times meaningful occupation touches the human spirit. At those moments, occupation becomes much more than its manifest task(s) or behavior.

The initial setting for next narrative is an urban shelter for homeless women. The setting then changes and the central figure, a resident named Julia, participates in an activity that has a profound effect on her well-being.

There are two references to possible clinical diagnoses impacting this resident: one is schizophrenia, the other is depression. However, we don't have the information to determine which may be more important in accounting for this woman's withdrawn behavior. Additionally, and perhaps most significantly, Julia is a woman who grieves.

"Julia" Narrated by Susy Stark, MSOT, OTR/C

The story that I'm going to share is about a client that I saw about a year ago. She is a 65-year-old woman who was diagnosed fairly early on, I think in her mid-20s, with schizophrenia. She came to us when she had been off her medication for about 6 months. She was fairly lucid at the time, considering how long she'd been off her medication. However, she also had a new onset of depression. Her two sons, who had been caring for her for the past several years, had been shot and murdered during some gang activity in their neighborhood. It was a rough area of the city. She had a daughter who lived in another state, who had a family of her own and was not interested in taking care of her mother. Eventually, Julia became homeless as a result of being unable to take care of her apartment and being unable to pay her bills. Basically, she had hung on in the neighborhood for a while, with no one saying much of anything, until she finally was evicted. She came through the homeless network to our shelter which specializes in caring for women with mental illness. When we first saw her, she was withdrawn and appeared very, very sad. She wore her hair in a turban and had a veil which covered her face. She reported that she used her veil as a symbol of her mourning for her children who were, as she said, "the most precious things" in her life to her. On evaluation, Julia demonstrated basic living skills that she needed to work on. She had been dependent on her sons for much of her care, not because she had been unable to care for herself, I suspect, but more because the boys respected their mother and felt that she had cared for them and they were going to do the same for her. When Julia came to us she was socially isolated, and hadn't had much community interaction for several years. During the past 6 months, she had been particularly lonely and had engaged in few of her former activities. Julia's goals were to develop some IADL (instrumental activities of daily living) skills that would allow her to live independently—budgeting, transportation, household management, and so on—in addition to raising her self-esteem and dealing with her feelings of hopelessness and loss. Projecting into the future, she described what she viewed as a potentially abysmal situation. At this point, she was fairly noncommunicative. She did not trust the staff. She spent her days mostly staring straight ahead while sitting at one of the dining room tables at the shelter, interacting minimally with the other residents.

In her therapy with me, the turning point for Julia came during a community outing. It was the second trip she had been on as part of her occupational therapy. She had agreed to attend this trip to the art museum along with several other residents, although she was reluctant. Up to this point, Julia had been quite noncompliant with her treatment. She was not meeting her specified appointments or attending the groups to which she was referred. Although her goals were to live independently, she had been unable to move toward those goals. Julia had expressed that she had enjoyed attending events at the art museum when she was younger and with her husband, but hadn't done so in several years. The primary goal in the outing was to work on residents' community reintegration and leisure skills. The secondary goal was to help them learn to use public transportation. In the beginning of the activity she was very reluctant, a definite follower. She required maximum assistance in following directions. Julia was able to follow two-step directions, but required prompting due to a lack of interest and motivation—hallmark signs of depression.

Julia, the other residents, and myself were wandering around the exhibits when she approached me to ask a question. This was unusual for her—she usually spoke only when addressed. Her speech was practically unintelligible. She spoke in a low mumble and it was very difficult to understand her. She was asking me about an exhibit, and a painting that she wanted to see. She mentioned the word "dancer," but I was having difficulty imagining what she was talking about. She became a bit frustrated with me, finally losing patience and walking over to the nearest security guard. I was amazed as this was quite a brave act for her, and totally out of character for what we had come to know of Julia. I watched as she explained patiently what she was looking for. The security guard nodded and indicated a direction that she should go and gave her some lengthy instructions. She came back to our group and asked us to follow her. We followed her through a difficult maze of rooms and spaces to reach the Impressionist gallery. I was astonished that she could have found her way and followed the directions, given her prior performance in the shelter.

She took us into the Impressionist gallery, and led us to a corner of the room where Degas' "Little Dancer" was on exhibit. She explained that this has been an important piece of work to her and that she had shared this experience previously with another person who had meant very much to her. She went on to say that this had been one of her favorite pieces of art since she was a little girl. All of this was quite a revelation. First, talking about her past had been very difficult for her. Second, there was by now a large group of us standing in the room giving Julia our full attention, and for her to share this in a public forum without prompting was even more startling. (As an aside, we were so rapt in our attention to Julia that I failed to notice that one of our other residents, Christy, had wandered off until several security guards came running from various sections of the museum. One took this woman by the arm and asked her why she was trying to pull the Monet off the wall. Christy later explained that she had been intrigued by the frame and was wondering how much it cost. She was just trying to look behind it to see what the price was.)

This incident marked a turning point in Julia's treatment. From then on she became much more active and involved with her therapy. She proceeded to achieve most of her goals for occupational therapy. She was successfully placed in housing with the help of the housing coordinator and moved into an apartment in the city where she now lives independently. It was symbolic, I think, that on the day she moved into her apartment she removed the veil from her face to begin a new phase of her life.

I feel the story is very powerful in the way that it demonstrates the meaning and symbolism that activity and community involvement can have. Julia went from being a closed and frightened woman to a blossoming older adult with some wonderful community ties and activities that she proceeded to pursue and enjoy.

Discussion Questions

1. When you read that this woman was homeless, what image did you get? Did anything in the story surprise you?
2. What do you know about the population of persons identified as homeless in your community?
   a. What resources are available for them?
   b. Is occupational therapy available to them? If so, in what settings?
   c. If not, what role do you see occupational therapy as having with homeless persons, and in what community settings might this best occur?
3. Describe in your own words what you believe happened with Julia at the art museum.
   a. How would you document this event for third party payers?
4. In what contexts have you seen the arts (i.e., music, dance) used as a therapeutic medium with clients?
   a. What has been the role of the arts?
   b. How do you see occupational therapy as a profession appropriately using the arts?
5. Have you ever been on a community outing with a client group?
   a. What were the goals of the outing?
   b. What, if any, concerns did you have regarding patient or client safety? How were these addressed by staff?
6. Propose and discuss a plan for providing staff supervision and communication during a community outing in which clients may scatter (e.g., a trip to a museum, a trip to the park).

Impressions

BB: As I first listened to this story, I keyed in on the words "schizophrenia" and "depression," and thought, "This woman will be placed on medication." And perhaps she was. Yet the breakthrough is not about medication. It is about engagement in meaningful occupation and about an essential yearning of the human spirit. Thomas Moore (1992, 1996) has written several books in which he talks about how beautiful music or other forms of art or nature can touch our lives. In his most recent book, he refers to these as magical or "enchanted" moments (Moore, 1996). When we work with people who seem confused or withdrawn, we most likely speak in terms of reality testing and not enchantment. It's almost as if we're afraid that if we touch their imagination, these people will go further away into their own thoughts and fantasies. I think it's very interesting that a work of art helped this individual reconnect.

The image of the veil and the eventual unveiling represent well what occurs in this story. Had the narrator been writing fiction, she couldn't have chosen a more suitable image or a more satisfying ending.

MAB: This story of therapy in a community context brings to mind numerous experiences I had during weekly community retraining (CRT) events while I was working in a day rehabilitation program. Clients participated in community outings to help them reengage in activities they had previously enjoyed and to decrease their social isolation, while practicing specific skills. I did not observe any dramatic changes such as the one Julia made, but weekly I saw clients meet the challenge of the community and verbalize pleasure and satisfaction in their achievements. The outings were planned by the clients themselves who looked forward to the treatment experiences with anticipation, enthusiasm, and sometimes fear of the challenge. From the therapist's point of view, I cannot emphasize enough the importance of good planning and being well-prepared for the unexpected. I learned to bring extra food for those clients who may forget to bring their lunch, and saw the benefits of having a portable phone for communicating with the hospital to advise them of traffic problems on the freeway or the van driver getting lost or client emergencies. Although we always carried an emergency kit, there are many events that don't require first aid, sunburn protection, or CPR masks, but require adequate staffing to provide supervision to ensure the safety of all participants. In most instances, everyone met their treatment goals, enjoyed the outing, and returned exhausted from the day's event. The CRT events helped patients to see their level of ability, broke the monotony of daily treatment in a rehabilitation setting, and helped clients and their families take new risks to increase their interaction in the community. Families, staff, and hospital administration recognized the value of CRT and supported the expense incurred for the program. Unfortunately, some third party payers developed the attitude that if a patient or client could tolerate these activities then perhaps they didn't need to be in therapy. Careful documentation and education of case managers was required to justify community treatment. However, very recently, given the current increased demand for productivity, the hospital no longer supports the staffing and time required for CRT. Therapists are educating family members to assume the responsibility for outings. Yet families and clients frequently need the support of staff presence before they are willing to take the initial risk of reentry into the community. And although I also did CRT in the context of the home care programs in which I worked, the benefits of a group CRT experience cannot be replicated in single-person community therapy. Clients in a group are motivated partially by the performance of others in the group. They take delight in sharing their accomplishments with other clients and benefit from group problem solving.

References

Moore, T. (1992). *Care of the soul: A guide for cultivating depth and sacredness in everyday life.* New York: Harper Collins.

Moore, T. (1996). *Re-enchantment of everyday life.* New York: Harper Collins.

CHAPTER 12

Awareness of Change

KEY TOPICS

- Alzheimer's dementia
- Anxiety
- Family denial
- Cognitive frameworks for occupational therapy practice
- Functional approach
- Dynamic interactional model
- Objects as cognitive organizers and links to identity and purpose
- Metacognition

Initial Comments

The main figure in our next story experiences a diminished sense of control due to cognitive decline. His response is anxiety, and as he becomes more anxious, his performance worsens. If we examine the therapeutic approach taken in this narrative, we see the application of many principles of a cognitive or cognitive-holistic framework and, with our attention given to cognitive approaches in occupational therapy, we make a few cursory comments. This story has themes similar to those preceding it, as we see the importance of objects in the client's environment. In this case, they not only provide comfort and a sense of identity, they seem to help organize his routine. We discern his need for control. Though the need to grieve is not directly addressed, it seems to dwell in the background, and we wonder about the family in this story. As in the previous story of Julia, this individual participates in an activity that has profound significance to him, and is equally moving to the narrating therapist. Echoing a theme repeated throughout the text, the therapeutic relationship is illustrated, as is the importance of helping the client maintain a sense of dignity and self-worth.

Cognitive Frameworks

Chapters 3, 8, 9, and 13 address various approaches to working with individuals with cognitive disorders. In our next story, several intervention strategies used are somewhat different than those discussed thus far. These strategies are described in occupational therapy cognitive rehabilitation literature.

In addition to Allen's model (Allen, Earhart, & Blue, 1992) and the behavioral approaches reviewed previously, occupational therapy literature identifies multiple cognitive models or approaches for assessment and intervention with persons having identified cognitive impairments, including those associated with neurologic disorders, mental disorders, and learning disabilities. The descriptions of cognition in these cognitive approaches suggest that the term "cognition" is used as a large umbrella. As used in the occupational therapy literature, the term cognition refers to "attention, orientation, perception, praxis, visual motor organization, memory, thinking operations, executive functions, problem solving, planning, reasoning, and judgment" (Katz, 1992, p. xii). Proponents of these cognitive approaches seem to agree that cognition underlies all human activities and occupations and influences one's health and well-being (Katz, 1992).

Kinds of Assessment

When comparing cognitive models within occupational therapy, Katz (1992) notes that a particular model may use formal assessment procedures (e.g., standardized, psychometric, and quantitative tests), naturalistic evaluation (e.g., functional evaluations, observation, interview, and other qualitative approaches), or a combination of approaches. Each model makes assumptions about cognitive impairment, one's potential for learning, the benefits of training, and the best methods for varying tasks and altering environments to facilitate successful function.

Dynamic Interactional Model

There are two additional cognitive approaches, themselves contrasting, that we review for the reader. The first of these is referred to as the dynamic interactional approach (Toglia, 1991, 1992, 1993). The other, itself comprised of a variety of strategies, has been called the functional approach (Toglia, 1992, 1993).

The dynamic interactional approach to cognitive rehabilitation is based on cognitive psychology theories of learning and is educational in thrust. It assumes that the individual is capable of learning, and that performance is influenced by (1) individual characteristics, (2) the type of task, and (3) the physical, social, and cultural environment. The interaction of these three factors is the focus of evaluation and treatment as suggested by the model's name (Toglia, 1991, 1992). To understand the interaction of these elements, this approach uses information processing and metacognitive theories along with occupational therapy principles.

Information Processing

Information processing theory describes a flow by which the person gets information (input) from the environment and then processes or elaborates information (via throughput) to produce an outcome (output). Obtaining information or input requires, in part, that the person explore the environment, initiate and attend to activity, manage multiple stimuli, and put together small pieces of information to create a broader, meaningful picture. When "processing" or elaborating information, the person contrasts and compares experiences and information, thinks about the incoming information, identifies problems in the current situation, forms and tests hypotheses, sets priorities, anticipates an outcome, and devises a plan of action. When one is able to process information to successfully bring about change, he or she also must engage adequate effort and energy to follow a plan to its completion, and must be able to tolerate the frustrations and distractions that arise during problem solving.

Metacognition

Metacognition is cognition about cognition. It implies that one knows how one learns best. When building metacognition, the therapist tries to help the client be more aware of his or her abilities, and the conditions that make it easier or more difficult for him or her to learn new information or skills (Flavell, 1985; Toglia, 1993, p. 23). An individual exhibiting metacognition, for example, might know about himself or herself, "I get distracted by the television or radio" or "I do better when trying new techniques hands-on" or "It helps me to write down (or say out loud or summarize to my spouse) the things I am trying to learn."

Dynamic Interactional Assessment and Intervention

When using the dynamic interactional model, the therapist evaluates the client's information processing strategies and the conditions in which he or she learns best. This knowledge can then be applied to many situations, rather than just one particular situation. If an individual has difficulty performing a task or learning information under a particular set of circumstances, rather than assuming that this person is globally incapable of performing the task, dynamic interactional assessment endeavors to determine what modifications in the task or the task environment might enable the person to succeed. For instance, the therapist might provide verbal cues to facilitate performance, or might dampen or strengthen stimuli in the environment, then note the nature and extent of these modifications. Cuing can then become a part of skill building, as illustrated in the story of Nathan (Chapter 9). The narrating therapist in that story describes cuing Nathan toward appropriate social and verbal responses to help him succeed.

A client's ability to generalize, or use his or her knowledge and skills beyond the rehabilitation setting, is evaluated. Using this approach, one goal in treatment will be to provide varied contexts or settings in which newly acquired skills can be practiced. Again referring to Nathan, the therapist has him practice self-control strategies at home as well as in a variety of social settings.

Intervention may be directed toward changing beliefs and emotional responses, for these, too, influence the dynamic person-system. In the following story, we learn that the client, Glenn, is anxious. If he could learn to monitor circumstances that heighten his anxiety and decrease his memory and performance, perhaps his task performance could be improved.

Therapists also evaluate individual characteristics and preferences which influence information processing and performance. It is believed, for instance, that people can more easily learn that information which they are motivated to learn (Toglia, 1993). Behavior patterns that interfere with (or enhance) learning across many tasks or situations will be identified (e.g., the tendency to be impulsive, to get overly focused on details, or to be self-critical). This information can then be used as the therapist helps the individual maximize his or her own learning.

Additionally, the therapist examines conditions in the environment to understand his or her influence on the client's thoughts, behaviors, and emotional responses. Within the social support system, for example, there may be one or more people whose encouragement can help the client function and learn. Conversely, one's peer group (e.g., a group of exuberant adolescents) may be distracting and undermine efforts at maintaining attention.

Function and Dysfunction

This approach does not attempt to classify cognitive function according to a number scale. The dynamic interactional model assumes that function changes as persons interact in their environment and learn. An individual is believed to be effective in the environment when he or she is aware of his or her cognitive capacity; can perceive, elaborate, and monitor information needed to function; and can flexibly use and apply the information.

Inadequate function results when the individual is unable to acquire and use information. Persons with cognitive impairments frequently overestimate their abilities, and therefore do not anticipate the problems they will have when they return to work or go home (Toglia, 1993). This may create conflict within families, as discussed further in Chapter 13.

Functional Approach

When the outcomes of intervention or the initial assessment data suggest that the patient is not capable of learning from a dynamic interactional (multicontextual) approach, Toglia (1992, 1993) recommends another kind of cognitive intervention: a functional approach. The functional approach assumes that the patient or client has limited ability for learning and transfer of knowledge and therefore uses domain-specific, adaptive, or compensatory strategies (Neistadt, 1990; Toglia, 1993, pp. 50-51). These strategies emphasize task performance rather than underlying cognitive processing skills (Toglia, 1993, p. 50). One type of functional approach is identified by Toglia (1993) as "adaptive" (p. 51). Caregivers change the task or aspects of the task rather than attempting to change the client. This philosophy is consistent with that described by Allen and the cognitive disability model (refer to Chapter 3). Citing an example given by Toglia (1993), if a client has difficulty remembering to wear all the clothing appropriate for a particular day, the caregiver might preselect the clothes and have them hanging and available to the client (p. 51). Adaptive approaches described in the following story include minimizing clutter and other distraction in the environment, and labeling the contents of drawers and containers so the client, Glenn, need not recall what has been placed in them.

Another type of functional approach is referred to as compensatory. In compensatory approaches, the affected client is required to change the way he or she goes about performing a task and must recognize the situation in which the strategy is to be used (Toglia, 1993, p. 52). For example, Glenn, in our next story, might be asked to follow up resident group meetings by writing the dates of upcoming events on his calendar. Or a client might be told to set an alarm to remind himself or herself that it is time to go to appointments.

Shared Strategies

The stories throughout this text have illustrated a variety of approaches used to respond to cognitive problems. In practice, these approaches may overlap and share techniques—for example, trying to increase generalization is consistent with behaviorism and Toglia's dynamic interactional approach. As you read about Glenn in our next story, think about which models or strategies you believe would be helpful for intervention with Glenn. As you consider his day-to-day performance, consider also the relationship and impact of his anxiety and other emotions on his well-being.

"Pagliacci" Narrated by Barbara Borg, MA, OTR

Glenn had cognitive dementia from Alzheimer's, and knowing him brought home to me what a cruel disease Alzheimer's is. He was a tall, lean gentleman, who stood erect and had a thick head of salt-and-pepper hair. When I saw him outside walking, he appeared just like the other walkers: healthy. Glenn was in his early 60s and had held a very responsible position during much of his life. Now he lived in a single room in an assisted living center where residents were carefully monitored by staff. His room was decorated with medals and commendations from his war experience and from work. He didn't remember his nurse's or my name, but he knew that picture on the wall was of Eleanor Roosevelt shaking his hand, and that she was thanking him. About the room there were signs of a strong Jewish faith. A displaced New Yorker, he told me once that he was still looking for a good delicatessen.

I was asked on two occasions to see Glenn. The first time, it was because he had stopped using his utensils properly at the common dining room, and the staff were concerned. As with many partial care living facilities, it was required that residents be able to manage the basics in living skills—dressing, eating, and bathing independently. Upon getting the referral, I asked myself, "Has this man forgotten how to use utensils, and if so, can I reteach him that, and will he forget again?" I didn't have to think about it too long as I soon received a call canceling the referral, with this explanation: "Glenn is incensed. He says he doesn't need any help from any occupational therapist in using a fork and knife!" (I later learned that he did need help but the staff decided to ignore protocol and cut his meat for him before serving it. The problem was, for the time at least, eliminated.)

The next time I was called, it was because Glenn had broken a window in his room. As best as the staff could determine, he had gotten a turtleneck shirt caught on his head in undressing, and had panicked. In flailing around, he had hit and broken the window. This time, the referral asked, "Could we simplify his room and routine" and thereby "decrease his anxiety." Anxiety seemed a significant problem for Glenn. Put simply, Glenn was aware that he was losing his ability for basic tasks, he could identify his disease by name ("I have Alzheimer's"), and he seemed to vacillate between reverie, denial, and tremendous fear. When he got anxious, his problem-solving ability decreased.

To get Glenn to agree to my visits, his caretakers and nurse decided to refer to me as an "ADL (activities of daily living) expert." The words "occupational therapist" were never used.

When I first met Glenn, we met in his room, and I could see where the need for simplification came from. There was stuff everywhere, especially papers—stacks of them—plus small pieces with notes to himself, all over the room. Interestingly, his grown son and daughter, who were both aware of the clutter, had resisted clearing the room for him. As his son said, "He likes to thumb through his papers. It's what he does every day for an activity." That took me aback for a moment, and I thought to myself, "Is that purposeful or purposeless activity?" I had several exchanges with Glenn's son and daughter and their consistent attitude was that their father was "scatterbrained," but otherwise not needing much extra care. I was so struck by this that I put a call in to the case manager to make sure that the family fully understood Glenn's condition and likely prognosis. She assured me that this had been discussed with the family on numerous occasions.

I was torn between not wanting to disturb Glenn's routine and seeing the need to get rid of some of the clutter. I decided to simplify. With the help of the family and with Glenn's permission, we removed nonseasonal clothes and anything else that was seldom used; mostly it was basic necessary items that were kept in his drawers, and these were kept exactly as he had them. Walls and decorations weren't touched. Some things were stored in his closet in labeled boxes. I brought him an 8" x 11" spiral notebook and suggested he take it with him everywhere and use it to write himself reminders. Overall, every effort was made to keep him from feeling that his belongings had somehow disappeared, and I tried to modify his routine as little as possible. When the room was in order, I asked Glenn how he liked it, half expecting that he would grumble, but he smiled and said, "I love it."

There was a particular interaction that most touched me. Glenn still loved opera and kept a collection of records in his room. (Those were not disturbed by the reorganization.) One day he asked if he might sing me one of his favorite songs. I'm unfamiliar with opera, but he told me the song was from *Pagliacci*. It was a poignant song, from the view of Pagliacci, a clown. Glenn closed the door to his room, then stood in the center of his room while I sat and listened. At first the song seemed to come easily to him, and he sang loudly, with a strikingly true voice. Then, in the middle, he abruptly stopped singing. It sounded like when the power goes off and a recording stops playing. He turned to me and said, "Please be patient with me. So many times people just walk away when I'm talking because I lose track of my thoughts, and when they do that, I feel so defeated. But if you give me time, I'll remember what it is I'm trying to say." Those were his words—he spoke that articulately. I sat and he stood silently for probably 4 or 5 minutes, and then he completed his song as if the power had been turned back on. When he was done, he beamed, and I thanked him, with a catch in my own throat.

Two weeks went by and I visited Glenn to see how he was doing. I walked into his room to see that scraps of paper and paper piles had begun to reappear.

Discussion Questions

1. What did you learn from the narrative?
2. Critique the decision of the therapist to declutter Glenn's room. With which cognitive model(s) does simplification of the environment fit?
3. What seems to be the role(s) of significant objects in Glenn's life?
4. How might you use Glenn's significant objects in your intervention with him?
5. In the narrative, the therapist writes, "scraps of paper and paper piles had begun to reappear." What do you conclude from this?
6. By what other means might you have tried to help Glenn manage his anxiety? Speculate on the utility of teaching Glenn relaxation techniques to cope with his anxiety. What additional information do you need before making a decision about relaxation training?
7. Try to put yourself in the place of Glenn's grown children. How would you feel? What would you fear?
8. What problems or issues would you like to have explored further if you were Glenn's therapist?

Impressions

BB: Glenn was my client and even now it's easy for me to picture him standing there in the middle of the room. Although I only had a handful of actual therapy visits, there was something in this moment that especially moved me. I wanted so much for him to be able to complete his song, and when he did, it felt like a huge victory for me also.

MAB: Reading this story about Glenn and reflecting back on the previous chapter in which we looked at how important objects are in everyday experience, I'm reminded of some of the ways objects can be used when working with persons who are confused or anxious like Glenn. With individuals who have traumatic brain injury and are difficult for staff to manage, I have heard families asked to bring in pictures of the patient prior to his or her injury, for instance, pictures with families, pets, or friends. These are placed on a bulletin board in the patient's room. They're used not only to help reorient the patient, but to serve as reminders to staff that this patient (who can be very hostile and aggressive) also has a history and another side that is much more engaging than the difficult person the staff works with daily. Bringing in favorite objects from the patient's home can serve the same purpose—these objects help humanize the environment and help us see the person inside the patient.

References

Allen, C.K., Earhart, C.A., & Blue, T. (1992). *Occupational therapy treatment goals for the physically and cognitively disabled*. Rockville, MD: American Occupational Therapy Association.

Flavell, J.H. (1985). *Cognitive development*. Englewood Cliffs, NJ: Prentice Hall.

Katz, N. (Ed.). (1992). *Cognitive rehabilitation: Models for intervention in occupational therapy*. Boston: Andover Medical Publishers.

Neistadt, M.E. (1990). A critical analysis of occupational therapy approaches for perceptual deficits in adults with brain injury. *American Journal of Occupational Therapy, 44,* 229-304.

Toglia, J.P. (1991). Generalization of treatment: A multicontextual approach to cognitive perceptual impairment in the brain injured adult. *American Journal of Occupational Therapy, 45,* 505-516.

Toglia, J.P. (1992). A dynamic interactional approach to cognitive rehabilitation. In N. Katz (Ed.), *Cognitive rehabilitation: Models for intervention in occupational therapy* (pp. 104-143). Boston: Andover Medical Publishers.

Toglia, J.P. (1993). Attention and memory. In C.B. Royeen, (Ed.), *AOTA self-study series: Cognitive rehabilitation*. Rockville, MD: American Occupational Therapy Association.

CHAPTER 13

Disability and the Family

KEY TOPICS

- Family dynamics and working with families
- Treatment planning and goal setting with families
- Traumatic brain injury
- Cognitive impairment
- Personality change
- Spousal abuse
- Establishing competence
- Return to work
- Return to home
- Driver training
- Financial management

Initial Comments

Not every client or patient we work with will have a family connection, but a great percentage do. If not actual family, there may be neighbors, coworkers, significant others, and friends who are the supporting cast in the life story woven by each client. As therapists, we may never meet these people face to face, but in many instances we affect their lives as much as we do that of our identified client. These people worry about their loved ones and about themselves; they call upon higher powers that this client might regain the ability to make a wage, pick up a child, take out the garbage, or respond to a hug. These people also can have what seem like unreasonable expectations, which make therapy and regaining function more difficult.

In physical rehabilitation and mental health settings, families and significant others may take on many responsibilities in the management of a particular patient or client. Family members learn to be caregivers through direct instruction in home programs, by observing therapists in therapy situations, or through educational and support groups for caregivers. Friends and family often are the primary emotional support for clients—the listening ear or the encourager. Family and friends may act as a language broker when the client does not speak the language of the health team. Family members, friends, or neighbors may take on additional responsibilities when clients cannot carry out their former roles. There are endless concerns that can weigh on all family members who wonder, "How will we manage?" Family and significant others understandably look to therapists for support, just like the client.

When, as therapists, we commence intervention with a client, we may be inclined to feel an allegiance to that individual. Sometimes, therapists become frustrated with family members or significant others who either hover too closely or fail to be supportive in carrying through with therapy programs. Often in our daily contact with the identified client, it is he or she with whom we can more easily empathize—for it is his or her "side of the story" with which we are more familiar. We might be wise, however, to remind ourselves that there are many versions of that story, and understanding the perspective of the whole family increases our ability to reach out in a manner that supports the entire family-as-client.

In our next narrative, we meet a male physician recovering from head trauma. We also meet his wife, who, through much of the story, appears as a nonsupportive, unappealing figure. As the narrative continues, we begin to realize why she may behave as she does, and the story moves from the all-good/all-bad depiction to one that illustrates the complexity of what goes on within a family.

There is a significant sub-theme within this story that relates to cultural values. This family identifies with a cultural group in which the man is traditionally the dominant figure, or "head of the house," as has been the case in this family. To protect the confidentiality of all people, we have chosen not identify this cultural group.

Additionally, this story illustrates some of the sequelae to head injury. The key figure, Dr. D., appears fully recovered physically, but has significant residual cognitive limitations and personality changes.

"Dr. D." Narrated by Mary Ann Bruce, MS, OTR

Prior to his head injury, Dr. D., a prominent physician, maintained one practice and was developing another in a distant part of the county. He was the father of three children, was active in his church and community, and saved one evening a week as date night with his spouse. His injury occurred on a mountain highway when a drunk driver hit his vehicle head on. He was unconscious for 3 weeks, with multiple internal injuries and a closed head injury. He was then hospitalized for about 3 months, first in intensive care, followed by treatment on an inpatient, acute rehabilitation unit.

I treated this client in an outpatient rehabilitation program. I quickly came to understand the frustrations that the acute rehab staff had communicated to our outpatient team. The frustrations were not regarding the client but his spouse. Documentation noted that Dr. D.'s wife was not adjusting to her current situation.

When visiting her husband, she usually left in tears. She verbalized some of her difficulties to staff but refused to see the psychologist when this support was offered to her. According to her, her "...total life had changed..." She now had financial worries, and she was "embarrassed" by her husband's behavior. Due to decreased inhibition, he now was jovial and outgoing, whereas he had previously been quite reserved. She indicated that she was having problems with two of their adolescent children who had begun to "act out" since their father's hospitalization. Also, in assuming responsibility for the financial management of the household, she learned about expenses of which she did not approve. Therefore, she was quite angry with her husband for what she viewed as his frivolous spending.

In their family, both partners viewed the man as the rightful head of the house. This was true also for the cultural community of which they were a part, and now was the first time in their married life that Mrs. D. had many of the responsibilities that she carried.

Not only did Mrs. D. refuse to see the psychologist, she infrequently attended monthly family conferences. She usually explained that she had another commitment or needed to respond to one of her children's needs. In the few meetings she attended, she sobbed throughout the session and left staff feeling conflicted about how to help meet her needs, address Dr. D.'s treatment needs, and solicit her assistance in problem solving. Early on, it was evident that she was unable to tolerate more stress than her current load at home. Some staff were able to empathize with her burdens but found it difficult to cope with what they described as "passive aggressive behavior," "sabotaging therapy," or "interfering with treatment goals."

The other thing that frustrated staff and led to an eventual dislike of Mrs. D. were the stories that Dr. D. would share during his treatment sessions. He described questionable, psychologically abusive treatment from his wife when he was home with her. After working with Dr. D., staff could be overheard discussing his stories, empathizing with his view that it was difficult to work with his wife to try to problem solve.

Staff continued to work with the woman to try to support this client's transitions into the community. To many of us as well as to the client, it seemed that no matter what he did, Dr. D. did it wrong. His wife seemed to be a perfectionist, which was reflected in her appearance, how she maintained her home, and her expectations for her children and for her spouse. She quickly became frustrated when her husband would forget to put away his medical journals, take out the trash, and so on. Over time, I realized that she viewed her husband's forgetting as being rebellious—"like an adolescent," she would say. I tried to explain that much of his behavior was an outcome of cognitive changes, but I couldn't discount that there might be a rebellious factor also.

When I spoke to Dr. D. about his memory problems and inability to follow the routine established for him at home, I soon deduced that while memory was a part of the problem, motivation was significant also. Dr. D. openly stated how much he "hated" doing things at home and in particular those things his wife decided. He wanted to have a choice; he intimated that he especially disliked that a woman was telling him what to do. Her view was that if given a choice, he would do nothing, or at least nothing that was needed. Also, Dr. D. verbalized that he could not see how competence in household responsibilities could prepare him to return to work. Returning to a part-time practice was his long-range goal.

Part of what Dr. D. worked on in therapy was increasing his physical strength and improving his body image so he could return to work. Physically, he made great progress, and 6 months after his accident there was little evidence that he had experienced major physical trauma.

The goal of returning to work produced many other dynamic problems. His physician and staff, and on occasion Mrs. D., met to analyze work tasks and establish a plan, and to evaluate ethical and legal considerations related to Dr. D.'s resumption of practice.

It became evident that the staff was enthused about the client's return to work, after all, if that was his goal, that was our goal. Mrs. D. never directly stated a reluctance for her husband to return to work, but set criteria the client should meet prior to his return to work. Sometimes the criteria were realistic; at other times, they seemed less so. In staff's estimation and as they described, she seemed to be setting up "barriers" for him. She expected him to remember and follow a routine at home, pick up the kids from school, fix dinner once a week, take out the trash, paint the bathroom, return to his scoutmaster responsibilities, and so on. The staff recognized that performance of these tasks could suggest competency, but they also knew that he had said he hated doing these things. He felt demeaned and, as he indicated, he did not want his wife "planning his life"; plus, he felt that he could "never please her."

In his physician's view, given the number of years the client had practiced, his foundation of medical knowledge was in his long-term memory. Doing routine procedures would not likely be a problem. His physician was concerned about Dr. D.'s ability to use this information and problem solve under stress. Would he be able to make accurate diagnoses? How might he respond in an emergency? Dr. D. exhibited a residual problem with self-monitoring—could this lead to distraction or making an error? Dr. D.'s physician was concerned for his client's accountability and also for his own if he was to sign an affirmation regarding Dr. D's ability to resume practice.

As the occupational therapist, I was identified as the person who would coordinate activities to foster Dr. D.'s eventual return to work. In addition to attending the previously mentioned meetings, I had the responsibility of making weekly phone calls to his spouse to get an update regarding the client's performance at home. After many telephone discussions, additional issues surfaced that needed to be addressed. Gradually, I became more aware of the problems Mrs. D. faced. The staff had focused primarily on the patient's competence for returning to work and on ethical considerations that would ensure that he could provide competent care. We had failed to consider the broader impact of his return to work on his family. In my telephone conversations with Mrs. D., it became evident that Dr. D. could never meet his current family financial demands if he returned to work part-time. His wife had adjusted the family financial budget to accommodate to the client's disability and insurance benefits—if he accepted disability pay and insurance compensation, the family could manage. These benefits would stop should he return to work even part-time. Thus, the dilemma she described was this: how can we provide financially for the family and still meet my husband's desire to return to work, if he can't work full-time?

She also spoke of their disagreements at home. This was not, she said, the "man I married." He was no longer the conservative, responsible partner she had made a life with—he was less inhibited and seemed like "one of the children." All this made me stop and think, "What must it be like to have someone change so much?"

Mrs. D. frequently brought up her husband's inability to manage his time. If he made a schedule, which he seldom did, he infrequently followed it. She liked making a schedule for him, which he detested. From my perspective, following Dr. D.'s accident, the dynamics between husband and wife had changed. Now she was the dominant partner, and she wasn't inclined to give this up. When I brought this time management issue to Dr. D.'s attention, he responded that in his office he had a secretary who made appointments and kept him on time when seeing patients. Therefore, he asked, why was this so important to him now? He didn't need to do this at work.

Given the circumstances, the team met to identify strategies that could act as interim steps to evaluate the client's cognitive competencies, meet some of his wife's expectations, and allow the client to work toward his goal. The outcome of the treatment team planning meeting was that Dr. D. would be asked to participate in professional continuing education courses which would provide professional contacts, and give him a means to update his knowledge and evaluate his ability for new learning. Dr. D. seemed to like this idea and he agreed to assume responsibility for finding short courses, registering for them, and taking any associated exams. Results would be shared with the team physician. This plan for continuing education was acceptable to Mrs. D., provided her husband didn't have family commitments and planned in advance. The next option identified by staff was for the client to provide medical services as a volunteer under the supervision of a physician, in a local clinic that provided free care for indigent patients. The client was to keep a log of his hours, the types of problems he treated, and the problems he encountered as a result of his head injury.

Dr. D. did not keep this log consistently. Instead, when he came for his outpatient occupational therapy session, he tried to recap verbally what he had done the previous week in his clinical practice. He stated that he did not like keeping the written log, that he was not convinced of its purpose, and he did not consistently remember to do it. I reiterated the functions of the log, which included tracking his own progress and providing concrete practice issues that he and his physician could examine.

He never did comply with our request for a log. His physician therefore refused to attest to his competence. One other option was suggested to Dr. D.—that he complete an internship under supervision. This, too, he refused and shortly after, he was discharged from outpatient treatment. From what I heard, he has continued to do volunteer work for the indigent, and continues to have marital problems.

Several months have passed and with the perspective I now have, I believe that as a treatment team we were too quick to see Mrs. D. as the "bad guy." She did some disagreeable things, but I'm not certain we fully appreciated how much she and the family had to cope with.

Discussion Questions

1. Give this story a new title and discuss what your title conveys.
2. With whom could you most empathize: Dr. D.? Mrs. D.? The occupational therapist? Dr. D.'s physician? The (unnamed) children in this family?
   a. Try to put yourself in the place of each of these persons and identify thoughts, feelings, or concerns you might be experiencing.
   b. What is it about this person or his or her role that you can identify with?
3. What factors do you believe most influenced the outcome of this story?
4. Are you comfortable with the manner in which goals were set with this patient and his spouse? Discuss other strategies that you think might have been helpful in responding to the concerns of both partners.
5. In this instance, the spouse (Mrs. D.) resisted speaking with the team's psychologist. Why might this have been?
6. Besides psychological counseling, what other resources might be available for spouses or children like Dr. D.'s?
7. If, as in this story, the occupational therapist and team believe spousal expectations to be unrealistic, what are some strategies that can be used to coordinate these with realistic treatment goals?
8. To what extent do you believe staff feelings might have influenced the events of this story?
9. To whom do you feel staff is responsible in this narrative? Discuss your answer.
10. How might cultural influences and values have affected intervention and interactions among client, spouse, and staff in this story?
11. Each team member might have some responsibility in attesting that Dr. D. is or is not competent to practice. As the occupational therapist, what behaviors, in the context of what specific activities, would you expect him to be able to perform that would indicate competence?
12. Are there specific assessment tools that you might use to determine competence?

13. When treating clients with a head injury, there are multiple issues to consider. Occupational therapists may assess a client's potential for return to employment, driving, and home management responsibilities.
    a. Identify the resources in your community for driver evaluation and training. If possible, gather information regarding their referral guidelines.
    b. Identify occupational therapy tasks or evaluations that can identify basic skills for return to driving and employment.
    c. Discuss what you view as the role of the occupational therapist in return to work evaluations and in job coaching.
    d. Discuss the issues that patients, family members, and therapists might need to consider when negotiating return to work, resumption of driving, and responsibility for finances.
    e. Identify issues that may be of concern to employers who support the client's return to work.
14. Indicate two behaviors (per role) demonstrated within activities that would indicate Dr. D.'s capability of resuming his other roles: father, spouse, and community participant.
15. Summarize what you see as the main issues in this story. Do you feel that they have been adequately addressed?

Impressions

BB: There is much to respond to in this story, but part of what remains unanswered for me is the extent to which staff feelings about Mrs. D. might have impacted her behavior, as well as Dr. D.'s, and perhaps fueled some of the ill will between husband and wife. As occupational therapists we might or might not be directly involved in resolving family tensions when we work with families. I know that on many occasions I've been asked by one or more family members to take their side in a dispute, or a client or a family member will use part of what I've said or part of a recommendation as proof that I'm in total agreement with him or her. That, of course, can create all kinds of problems. I try to remind myself that clients don't necessarily share the same information with every staff member or care provider that they come into contact with. Therefore, each of us may get a different piece of a picture. Probably, we both knowingly and unwittingly encourage clients and family members to share particular kinds of concerns with us. And each of us, having our own personalities, can get hooked by certain issues close to our hearts. Whatever our involvement, I believe that once we have entered the family's story, we will influence its outcome.

Whether it's the man or the woman who is dominant in a couple relationship, as therapists we often see striking changes in couple and family dynamics as each family member takes on (or gives up) particular roles. That can be tremendously stressful. I've seen evidence of physical abuse on several occasions.

In one instance I remember, the husband was very frustrated with his wife's inability to assume her usual responsibilities in the home and was reported to have begun hitting her in the head with the telephone when he became angry with her. Both partners abused alcohol also.

In another instance, the wife of my client would wheel her husband into their garage and leave him there for extended periods. As she said, she couldn't bear to look at him "...just sitting there, doing nothing, saying nothing." In the first example, we contacted Social Services and they acted to protect the wife. In the second, I alerted the case manager and we all worked with the wife to teach her tools that she could use to better cope and communicate. With neither of these couples was it a clear case of villainy, as it might sound. The spouses in both these instances had significant physical and emotional problems themselves.

As therapists, and people, we are not super-human, and I'm sure that we often are more sympathetic to the concerns of a particular individual in a family, even if we're trying to be fair. This narrative reminds me that in most stories of therapy, there are many characters. Each would tell the story a bit differently.

MAB: This story raises a concern I have frequently experienced in the settings in which I have worked: how to adapt occupational therapy, or rehabilitation in general, to meet the needs of persons who are extremely competent and high achievers. Frequently, they have achieved a great deal in life, have been in powerful positions at home and in the office, are recognized in the community for their achievement, and have been earning a relatively high wage. All this influences how they perceive activity, and their expectations for themselves and for treatment. As I think about how we as staff responded to Dr. D., who was a high achiever, I am choosing to respond to three particular areas in this story: staff empathy, family dynamics, and the impact of this patient's career and social status on his recovery and rehabilitation. Then I would like to further address some of the skills that need to be considered before a client returns home.

In this story, staff's empathy for the patient decreases their awareness and sensitivity to family dynamics, family history, and the impact of the trauma and disability on the entire family. Although I know trauma affects the family, I must admit I had a limited sense of the impact until one day a woman commented to me about her husband, saying "This is not the man I married." That was many years ago and, since then, I have heard this comment frequently from husbands and wives who are coping with the impact of trauma. I feel this statement gives insight into the amount of change with which families cope. Staff members can't know how the family feels, in part because they have little or no previous knowledge of the patient/client, and therefore have fewer expectations. Although family meetings may solicit information and establish rapport and a working relationship with families, these meetings can provide only a limited view of the extent to which the patient's personality and function have changed, and the day-to-day impact of the disability.

Given that staff have more frequent contact with clients or patients than family members, it may be easier for staff to empathize with patient concerns than with family members'. As a result, on some occasions I have seen staff assume that the family member is sabotaging treatment when he or she fails to support staff recommendations or patient desires. And even though I probably have made similar assumptions, I'm not sure I really know what "sabotaging" entails, and doubt if most families intentionally interfere with treatment. My experience with Dr. D. and his family reminded me of the need for a broader understanding of family dynamics, and led me to renew my commitment to soliciting and listening to the family's perspective.

The work with Dr. D. also reminded me of other changes that an individual copes with following trauma. Dr. D. had a huge loss of power and prestige. Even though we tried to praise his accomplishments in therapy, this couldn't take the place of the professional prestige typically given to physicians. Patients and clients may hesitate to change their behavior, because the change affects their self-image as well as life satisfaction. It may be hard, for example, for someone used to being in charge to now be taking orders, or for someone used to being very independent to have to ask for guidance. Usually, these changes serve as frequent, painful reminders of the losses the patient has incurred due to trauma. Thus, individuals who appear uncooperative, like Dr. D., may not be avoiding responsibility as much as they are avoiding a painful confrontation with the physical and psychosocial loss accompanying disability.

While this story focuses on establishing whether or not Dr. D. would be able to resume work, therapists who help clients prepare to return home may assess or refer for assessment additional areas of functioning, such as driving, child care, or financial management.

In the neurorehabilitation outpatient setting in which I saw Dr. D., one of the first questions usually asked by patients was, "When do I get to drive?" I always responded with, "Your doctor makes this decision." I then described the role of occupational therapy in these decisions. In the outpatient setting, during treatment sessions, the patient would participate in activities that provided information about his or her performance in skill areas needed for driving, work, financial management, child care, and others. Information regarding the patient's performance would be shared with the patient, family members, and physician. In the case of driving, I also described to patients and family members the resources available for driver assessment and training, when the patient was ready for these programs. The reader is referred to the occupational therapy literature in the area of driver assessment (Cook & Semmler, 1991; Galski, Bruno, & Ehle, 1992; Galski, Ehle, & Bruno, 1990) for detailed descriptions of these assessments.

Although a driver training program was not available in the outpatient clinic where I treated Dr. D., we frequently made referrals to a driver evaluation and training program in another county. This program provided us with a guide specifying basic skill prerequisites for driving success. We used this guide to test and evaluate these skills, such as attention, reaction time, and visual motor function. We made recommendations to the physician when the patient could demonstrate basic skills. We also gave patients opportunities to practice the written driver test. Even when patients felt ready to take the driving test, their families were not always in agreement. In those instances, we often recommended the driver evaluation program because of its extensive skill evaluation and because they used tests in the "real world" (e.g., on the freeway). This and other driver evaluation and training programs usually have worked with state Department of Motor Vehicle (DMV) departments. Driver assessment and training programs usually meet the guidelines of the DMV. Therefore, they are a good assessment of potential readiness for the patient to go to the DMV for testing. This sometimes increased family confidence in the patient's performance, but did not necessarily influence the family's decision to allow the patient to return to driving. In the case of Dr. D., he wanted to resume driving, and successfully completed the driver retraining program. However, Mrs. D. refused to ride in the car with him, and wouldn't allow their children to be driven by him.

When working in an area that involves safety, it is important to work with family members (and employers, if the client returns to work) to inform them of the client's abilities and limitations and possible resources, and to solicit their agreement as to goals that have been established. This process often requires education of family members and employers. Therapists must be sensitive to family concerns. Family members may be fearful for the patient as well as the safety of others, and may be anxious about legal implications should auto accidents, poor work performance, financial errors, or child abuse occur.

The occupational therapist bases recommendations on skilled performance as well as the contexts in which the skills are safely demonstrated. For example, clients may be able to perform work tasks in the clinical environment, but with stimuli in the actual workplace, frequent interruptions, or expectations for high productivity, the patient may be unable to meet work requirements and problem solve. Therefore, job coaching in which work tasks are negotiated with an employer—and in which the therapist participates in the employment setting and assists the patient with problem solving—can provide the support and feedback required for return to work.

The difficulty with living alone, returning to work, and driving is that the patient often has extensive experience, and therefore, much of his or her performance is automatic. As a result, patients frequently are convinced that they can care for themselves, drive, and do their jobs. I have spent much time explaining to them and their families that the issue is not just performing the task but the conditions under which they will be able to do the tasks safely.

Even when patients are ready for and capable of increased independence and responsibility, family members do not always support goals and therapist recommendations. For example, when teaching financial management, a task frequently practiced in occupational therapy, I became aware of family members' discomfort with patients working toward independence in this area. They feared patient error, or sometimes, they liked having control of this area of household management. In these situations, I usually evaluated the patient's competency and advised both patient and family of the patient's ability—they then determined how responsibility would be handled. One caution: even when patients can do financial tasks competently, it doesn't necessarily mean that they can monitor when bills are due or do related planning. Also, we know that just because a patient can perform under clinical conditions does not mean that he or she can perform in other contexts. It is advisable to test performance in varied environments.

References

Cook, C.A., & Semmler, C.J. (1991). Ethical dilemmas in driver education. *American Journal of Occupational Therapy, 45,* 517-522.

Galski, T., Bruno, R.L., & Ehle, H.T. (1992). Driving after cerebral damage: A model with implications for evaluation. *American Journal of Occupational Therapy, 46,* 324-332.

Galski, T., Ehle, H.T., & Bruno, R.L. (1990). An assessment of measures to predict the outcome of driving evaluations in patients with cerebral damage. *American Journal of Occupational Therapy, 44,* 709-713.

CHAPTER 14

Client Perceptions

KEY TOPICS

- Changes in self-perception
- Personal standards
- Depression
- Traumatic brain injury
- Grounded theory
- Adjusting to disability
- Community reintegration
- Community treatment programs
- Dependence
- Family education
- Individualizing treatment
- Performance feedback
- Journaling
- Spousal support

Initial Comments

Unlike the other stories in this text, told by occupational therapists, this next story is told by a client. Kevin shares several entries from his personal journal which together create a story he entitled "Life as a Disabled Person (1993)." Kevin, now 32 years old, became disabled after he was in an accident in which the car he was driving was broadsided by a vehicle that ran a red light. As a result of the trauma, he had multiple physical injuries and was unconscious for 6 weeks. He was in intensive care for 3 months, followed by many more months of hospitalization, then rehabilitation. He has residual physical limitations, which include being left with 50% lung capacity and residual cognitive disabilities. In his story, Kevin provides a perspective on disability and rehabilitation over a 3-year period. He also identifies his "Rules for Living," or what he more recently refers to as "Kevin's Antidepression Drugs (1993)." Kevin's journal and his "Rules" were given to Mary Ann Bruce following a weekly support group meeting, in which he participated and she led. At that time, he indicated that he was interested in having his material published someday. Kevin had attended the adjustment group for about 1 year, and frequently shared his experiences and perceptions with other group members, who also had disabilities subsequent to head trauma or neurological diseases and disorders. The group met weekly to problem solve and provide support for managing ongoing problems which members experienced in daily life.

When we contacted Kevin about including his story in this book, he replied that he was honored, and added that he would need to edit his work prior to publication because "it's probably not very good." We explained to Kevin that we felt his story represented a stage in his recovery and that he probably had changed; therefore, we encouraged Kevin to write an addendum to his story rather than edit it. We also invited his wife, Polly, to share her perspective on the therapy experience, should she and Kevin wish.

Kevin's journal entries from 1993, his "Rules for Living," and an addendum from 1996 are printed as written with his permission. Typographical errors, sentence structure, and spelling have not been edited. Polly's response also is published as written with permission. After each of the story components—the 1993 entries, the 1996 addendum, and Polly's piece—we pose questions and give our impressions just as in the other chapters of this text.

"Life as a Disabled Person (1993)" Journal by Kevin

It is certainly difficult to deal with the fact that you are now and for the rest of your life, a complete moron. What makes it more difficult is that you remembered that you were once someone important. You've had a title, a promising career, a killer educational background and a good life. When you were in college, and you were struggling, everyone cheered you up by saying "Once you got your degree and your education no one, absolutely no one can take it away from you". Well I proved that theory wrong.

Professionals in the disabled field such as doctors, nurses, therapists, health instructors, etc...are conditioned not to have the word "never" in their vocabulary. There are always exceptions. However, sometimes one has to be realistic. When I was a design engineer, the tasks were mostly complex and lengthy. Patience, organization, as well as creativity were essential. With thousands of qualified engineers out of work, it is very safe to say that "convincing a potential employer that I am the right person for an engineering position with my deficits in those areas above", is a slim to none opportunity. In this uncertain world we live in, it is just about the only sure thing, that I will probably not return to the engineering field. Maybe I came from the wrong end of the totem pole. However, I do believe that the term "Mild Head Injury" does not ever apply. I believe that "Traumatic Head Injury" applies to every case. It definitely is a traumatic experience to every victim. Everyone knows that a head injury has devastating effect on every facet of the victim's life. Even a moron can figure this out.

Therapists have always told me to look on the positive side of an issue whenever I get frustrated. Initially, after my injury (through the first two years), I always looked at the "glass half full. I compared myself with others having similar injuries at rehab, hospitals, (...name of program) THI program, and so on. I felt so fortunate of my situation that things could have been far worse and it was not. I had great family support, my cognitive thinking abilities were still in good connection, therefore, life was rosy. However, the closer I became to my old-self, the more I started to realize how many things that I had lost and that I could no longer do. Activities such as basketball, skiing, running, pool-shark, softball are still missing. It seems so easy to say "learn them again, keep practicing, and things will improve". Mentally, it is very difficult to initiate the activities that you once had no trouble of mastering. Doing these activities inevitably puts me back into depression. I have found that the best defense against depression is to avoid these activities all together. I have long stopped feeling sorry for others with disabilities because I've lost so much also. This may seem selfish and harsh but it puts reality into proper perspective. In conclusion, the catch-22 about recovery is that the closer you become to your old-self, the farther the distance to being your old-self. Am I making any sense here?

Most victims of severe disabilities cry out the same message. They do not want sympathy. Empathy and an understanding ear around them is all it takes to turn their attitude around 180 degrees. What they are really looking for from their families and peers is a lot of patience with them.

The moral to the story here is that life is a mystery, and one must not take the things that he/she does well for granted for things can quickly change path. Since my injury, I have learned to live life everyday to its fullest. If for some reason I knew ahead of time that I only have a few days to live, I would not have any regret that I have not done "so and so" not and would be in a hurry to finish any unfinished business, because I'm living life to its fullest thus far.

Positives of Being a Disabled Person

Obviously, the picture isn't as grim as I painted above. If it is, suicide might not be a bad option. Seriously, I don't think anyone with a disability has not contemplate the option of suicide. Any disabled person that tell you anything different is simply not being truthful. My mental outlook about this situation is so simple. The man upstairs has chosen me to get a second chance for whatever reason unknown to me, as of this time. It would be a tragedy to waste this chance on something studpid. Furthermore, things just have a habit of working themselves out, no matter how hopeless the situation may look at the time. One just has to trust this fact.

If one is fortunate enough, his/her doctors might give a prescription for a permanent disabled parking placard. The benefits are limitless. Not only are you pretty much untouchable to parking tickets, "except for red-zones", you don't have to pay in metered zones. At service stations, the clerks have to pump you gas, give you full service treatment at self-service prices.

Besides the practical benefits, there are a few intangible factors as well. Certainly, one of the things you immediately notice is that people, in general, are eager to give you assistance if you ask. They will open and close the doors or get things for you. At the very least, they are generally more pleasant toward you. Certainly you will quickly realize your true friends, the ones who will stand by you no matter what your disabilities. In a madness world we live in tainted by mostly by the media, this fact suddenly gives you hope for humanity and mankind.

The one factor that really stand out is the fact that my character was certainly shown up. Let me provide an example to clarify this point. In the summer of 93, I volunteered at a trauma center (my alma-mater). Late one night, I was consoling a lady whose son was in a coma from an automobile accident. "Why do bad things happen to good people" she asked me. I was momentarily lost and desperately searching for an answer. Finally I told her "bad things happen to everyone, and good people are not immune". "And God wanted it to happen this way" I added. "How so? she replied as she was obviously confused. "Characters appear only in rough conditions, when a storm hits and the ocean is swelling, not in calm smooth sailing" I responded. The one positive experience about this injury is that I know I have the right character to face the next challenge. The one constant in life, and a reward for good recovery, are more challenges are sure to happen with life. More difficult situations are sure to rise. I now know that I have the necessary character to face them.

Everyone with a handicap must, in every facet of his daily living, make some sort of adjustment. Adjustment is needed for everything from memory to organizational skills to some sort of physical ailments. A different sort of adjustment which I feel is too important to go unnoticed is the adjustment of daily activities of the disabled. Before my injury, I would wake up every morning with a list of "things to do" for the day, all in my head. By the end of the day, most of the items would be checked off. Presently, one of my biggest surprises which required so much mental adjustment, is this list of "to do's". Since the injury, I still have the list every morning, but by the end of the day, I am exhausted and I still have more than half of the list to go. The effort is there, it is just that I cannot be like my old self and accomplish these tasks in the allotted time. The unfinished business on this list is a constant reminder that I have a disability. It reaches out and slaps you on the face every time you get the idea that you are improving and nearing your old self. Certainly, you have to maintain your mental outlook despite the disappointments. Personally, this is by far the toughest mental adjustment to date in dealing with my disability.

Recovery

I may not be a certified Physical, Occupational, or Speech therapist nor do I claim to have any experience or schooling in such fields. From my observations in my recovery, I can make the following conclusions. One aspect that frustrates or aggravates professionals in such fields is the lack of one single universal method of treatments for all individuals. Everyone recovers at their own unique pace and finds each type of treatment unique to of their own beneficial. One type of treatment may work very well for one person or group, but not others. This lack of standardize method forces therapists to be creative when it comes to choosing to rehabilitation techniques. However, there is one common method of rehabilitation which somewhat resembles universal. A unique to mankind which is "learning from mistakes". Therapists just learn to supervise the rehabilitation method and put safety under consideration before beginning the sessions, then let mistakes happen. The disable patient will quickly learn from those mistakes and improves. AAAhhh, the beauty of nature.

My Experience at (...name of institution) Community College

In November 1993, I started at (name of college) Head Injury program. (Name of college) Special Programs pride itself as the only rehab facility of its kind, to cognitively rehabilitate the head injury cases of stroke victims. On paper its a worthwhile program. I could join the majority who have said that this was a wonderful experience, and so on. Being the exception, I feel that I must share the actuality from my personal perspective. Like everyone else, I've had my share of ups and downs with many subjects, staff, personal life, and so on. Half way through the program I was not enjoing life as I should. One of the main frustrations of disabled individual is trying to convince others that you are capable and competent at certain subjects. The stereotype of "disabilities" somehow reaches to distrustful. People, especially professionals, just do not trust the competency of the disabled. I guess my biggest criticism about (name of college) personnel is all too common with the media. It seems that they put too much focus on deficits, not accomplishments. In addition they (the staff) are obsessed with the idea that no one is above anyone else. It is as if there flat line on the X-Y graph where everyone lies on the line with no one above anyone else. The traditional "Gaussian" curve is nonexistent. Public appraisals or acknowledgment on exceptional instances or performance comes just about as often as the occurrence of the "blue" moon. I must also give credit where credit is due, with constant associations with the disabled all day, the staff developed pretty clear instincts. The down fall about these instincts is that they tend to generalize specific individuals lumb them into groups and unjustly label them. Furthermore, their personal preference with certain subject matters further clouds the picture. God forbid if your opinion is in conflict with theirs. In my personal opinions this program is no different then any other state run program.

The program does benefit those that are left severely disabled by their injury to the point that they are dependent on others for their daily activities and simple decision making. In such cases, the staff can flex the muscles and apply their controlling influences on such individuals. The results are surprising beneficial. For cases where individuals recovered well or less handicapped by their injury, these people are more independent to their actions and decisions. In these particular cases, the methodological belief applied here may actually digress the results for individuals.

However, I've learned to put aside my frustrations and live day by day. Furthermore, I've learned to trust the fact that, as I said above, "things somehow just have a habit to falling into places. After all, they are humans too.

Moving Ahead

As I stated earlier, we as humans main goal in life is to improve and stretch our limits at whatever we do best. Humans cannot stay in the same arena for very long. No difference to the disabled population. Simply state, the disabled people all want to recover and getting back to employment, where he/she was previously. There is no incentive to sit around and collect S.S.I. There are some do's and don'ts when it comes to recovery to an employment career. First and foremost, due to memory and learning challenges, the handicapped really should consider returning to the field where he previously was employed. In this way he has familiarity with the subject. After a traumatic experience, the victim always has different perspective on life in general. The temptation to try something new is overwhelming. There is always an exception, that his can be successfully be accomplish but this is not a good idea.

The subject of disclosure is always a difficult one for the disabled. In my particular advise, there are three audiences of disclosure, the immediate Supervisor or Manager, the work mates, and causal friends. First, prior to employment, disclosure to potential employer should be on the basis of "Don't ask, Don't tell", unless your deficits are in direct requirement of the position. For example, you should not hide the fact that you have memory problems for Air Traffic Controller position. If the interviewer does not ask any questions, don't feel obligated to tell give them more ammunition. There is no need give the potential employer reasons "not to hire you". It is a very competitive world out there. The employer has to fulfill the bottom line, keep worker comp's cost at a minimum, oblige to the A.D.A. After getting the position, it is a good idea to disclose to your immediate supervisor. Some of the mistakes that you might make may not be taken out of context with your honesty. For workmates and causal friends, the decision is up to the individual. True friends will emerge from the causal friends crowd upon the knowledge of disability. Work mates disclosure may not ne a good idea. As an employer, I despised the fact that there were always some type of conflict among employees. Employers do not want to choose sides and remain impartial. Disclosure to other work mates may eventually lead to some sort of discontent or disagreement and the injury is almost always the source for the blame.

Be prepared and organized and detailed as much as you could possibly be. Write out the game plan and keep referring to it. Remember, repetitions may hold the key to a job well done. Don't leave too little time for a task so there is the pressure to rush. Most likely, you will not have the patience to conquer this emotions. More importantly, if you are stress out, put off the project until later when you've got a clear head. More importantly, never drive when you are stressed out. The mind of the disabled does not work nearly as well when the situation becomes foggy with stress.

Advises for the Disability to Live a More Balanced Lifestyle

My health crisis was Nov. 1992. Thus I've had much time to reminist and reflect on the situation. I've got just a few tips for those unfortunate souls who joined disabled population. First and foremost, one should seek a spiritual side among themselves. I think it is very important to seek a spiritual guide to give some kind of hope and guidance to a senseless situation. Secondly, I could not stress further the importance of an old cliche, well known to the medical community. That is "Take life one day at a time". Think about it. There isn't much we can do about the events yesterday. There isn't much in life that we have control with. Therefore, we certainly cannot do much about tomorrow's events. Every morning, one should view his day as a new opportunity. If he seize the opportunities presented to him today, he will give himself much better odds for having a good day tomorrow. Finally, one last tip for a balance life. The medical field has much giant leaps of progression the last 20-25 years. One field that I would like to see more research in is the "effect of humor on the immune system". Certainly, when we laugh, we do not exhibit any critical symptoms, such as high blood pressure, heart rate, etc.. Everyone should find their funny bone and give into laughter a few times a day.

"Kevin's Antidepression Drugs (1993)" (Original Title—"Kevin's Rules for Living") Journal by Kevin

"There" Is No Better Than "Here"

When you finally get "there", you will be "here". You will once again find another "there" that will once again look better than "here". It is an infinite loop with no better place. Think about it.

What You Make of Your Life Is Up to You

You have been borned with all the tools and resources you need. What you do with them is up to you. The choice is yours.

You Will Learn Lessons

You are enrolled in a full-time informal school called life. Each day in this school you will have the opportunity to learn lessons. You may like the lessons or think them stupid.

Learning Lessons Does Not End

There is no part of life that does not contain lessons. As long as you are alive, there are lessons to be learned.

Forget the Daily Drugs and Medication, Give Your Immune System a Daily Dose of Humor

When your are laughing and having a good time, your vital signs (blood pressure, heart rate, etc.) can't be very high. Much more research needs to be done on the relationship of humor and one's immune system.

Worry About Jumping of the Bridge, When You Get to It!

We cannot undue the events of yesterday. There are very few things in life that we have control over. Therefore the events of tomorrow are uncertain, at best. We should seize the opportunities of todays' events to give ourselves a better chance for a good tomorrow.

Slow Down! Use All Your Senses and Absorb the Environment

Life is meant to live as "frame by frame", not as a "blur". Remember, it is always better to be late in this lifetime than early for the next.

When You Find Yourself in a Bind, Tell the Truth

Give your brain a break. Less brain cells are needed to remember one truth versus keeping tract of many lies.

These Drugs Are Nice But You Will Forget All This

Discussion Questions

1. Identify and discuss three questions regarding recovery and living with a disability.
2. How did Kevin see himself before his head injury? Identify the changes you see in Kevin's self-image since his accident.

3. Summarize in your own words how Kevin views health professionals and professional practices.
4. Describe situations where you perceived health professionals behaving in a manner either similar or dissimilar to that described by Kevin.
5. Think about Maslow's hierarchy of needs. Which level of need is Kevin trying to meet?
6. Does it appear that Kevin's values have changed since his injury? If so, in what way?
7. Kevin states that he wants to live life to its fullest. What does this appear to mean to Kevin?
   a. What would this mean to you?
8. If you could talk with Kevin, what questions would you like to ask him after reading his journal?

Impressions

MAB: When Kevin gave me his story following the Adjustment Group, he asked for my impressions. I briefly shared my reactions and my belief that students could learn from his descriptions of his recovery following a head injury. About a year later, in a doctoral seminar for theory development, I used the principles of grounded theory to study "Life as a Disabled Person (1993)" and "Kevin's Rules for Living."

Grounded theory (Glaser & Strauss, 1967; Strauss & Corbin, 1994) is a qualitative research methodology used to develop theory directly from the analysis of verbal or written narrative data or video documents. When analyzing the data, the researcher identifies relationships and recurring themes to gain a scientific understanding of "real world" phenomena over time. The analysis is influenced by the subject's and the researcher's unique views on life (Strauss & Corbin, 1994, pp. 273-285). For example, in this chapter, we make comments about Kevin's narrative based upon our own interests and values. When you read the narrative, you may see different themes and relationships than those we discuss.

When I used grounded theory to understand Kevin's story, many themes and relationships emerged. Of these, three influence my comments here: change and the pain of recovery, the effect of control and choice during recovery, and the influence of health care professionals on the attitudes and beliefs of the client.

The changes in Kevin's skills, leisure interests, and employment opportunities affect his emotions and interactions with others. These changes also influence his willingness to return to previous occupations or participate in adapted activities. Kevin describes the pain of recovery when he states that he feels "slapped on the face" each day when he is unable to finish all of his planned activities. When he no longer can perform some activities, the meaning of the task changes, along with his level of interest. Therefore, he gives up some occupations and develops new interests. He states, "Mentally, it is very difficult to initiate the activities that you once had no trouble of mastering." Therefore, he wishes to avoid activities such as basketball, skiing, running, and playing pool.

Kevin not only avoids previous leisure interests, he also is aware of a need to change (or modify) his work responsibilities. He is unable to meet his previous performance standards and is aware of being unable to meet the expectations of others. He feels that he will not be able to return to engineering. As he recovers, he looks for meaningful occupation and explores the volunteer role. In his description of volunteer work, we learn that Kevin, like many clients, finds meaning in the opportunity to contribute to the welfare of others rather than just receive service. In this role, Kevin provides support to others experiencing trauma, and feels good about his contribution. He also can test his current abilities and get feedback regarding his performance outside of the rehabilitation program. Volunteer experiences can support Kevin and other clients in recovery and transition to a work role.

Kevin's story addresses various control issues. Like all of us, he wants to have control, and sometimes, he chooses to give up control. He evaluates the extent of his control daily, and sometimes gives up control to a higher power and trusts that "...things just have a habit of working themselves out, no matter how hopeless the situation..." Here, Kevin refers to spiritual beliefs and their role in recovery and coping with disability. Like Kevin, I have heard other patients speak about a higher or greater power outside themselves that gives them strength and hope.

Kevin describes his loss of control when he says that there are "...few things in life that we have control over..." I frequently sense this feeling of diminished control from people who experience trauma. They have lost physical ability, social and financial status, had their daily routines disrupted, and experienced other losses that bring about depression and economic stress as well as a sense of loss of control. Helping patients regain a sense of control is one challenge of therapy.

In the story, Kevin suggests that health care professionals and family members influence his sense of control, and he asks that they provide an "understanding ear" which can turn the patient's "...attitude around 180 degrees." He asks for "empathy," and for staff to have "realistic" expectations. He wants to be treated as an individual, and he wants staff to remember that there is no "...one single universal method of treatments for all individuals. Everyone recovers at their own pace." Kevin's story reminds staff to consider patient opinions when negotiating treatment goals and activities, and to give positive feedback regarding performance along with constructive recommendations for change. He wants to be recognized for his accomplishments and given guidance based on realistic expectations for his future performance.

When thinking about his future and return to work, in the section "Moving Ahead," Kevin describes a concern that I have heard many times. Patients are conflicted about what information to share regarding their accident, injury, or illness, and whom to inform. I cannot agree with his views on disclosure which he summarizes with "Don't ask, Don't tell." I do, however, agree with the criteria he says to consider: the person (e.g., friend, boss, colleague), the content, and the timing of the disclosure. In general, disclosure is a topic patients and clients need to discuss with their family, physicians, and therapists. Individual guidelines on what to disclose, the extent of detail to reveal, and to whom to disclose can be decided within the context of the individual's circumstances. Patients discuss this topic among themselves, and occupational therapists can be active participants, providing moderating views and helping patients see the consequences of their choices.

In summary, every time I read Kevin's story I increase my understanding of Kevin's recovery and am reminded of the connection between mind and body during recovery and of similar concerns from other clients who are coping with the outcomes of head trauma.

BB: What struck me in Kevin's story is the extent to which he measures himself and his performance. He writes about having a list of things to do but, at day's end, still has "more than half of the list to go." And although he feels bad that he can no longer meet the performance standards he sets, he expresses dismay that the helping community too often lumps (the disabled) into groups and seldom acknowledges "exceptional instances or performance." He dislikes that staff place clients on a "flat line" rather than a "Gaussian curve." There are many descriptions that allude to measurement, but the one that captures it best, for me, is when he writes that, "the closer you become to your old-self, the farther the distance to being your old-self." What he says, in a sense, is that he will never measure up, and we see this through the rest of the journal.

The extent to which we measure or establish standards, what we choose to measure, and the yardstick we select depends on what each of us values. Kevin's yardstick is rigid, and appears to lack the middle numbers: one either measures "0" or the full "36 inches." Kevin indicates that he values intellect, independence, formal education, and top-notch performance. He also appears to value spirituality, and struggles now to value day-to-day experience where accomplishing longer term goals had formerly motivated him. When I read Kevin describe himself as "now and for the rest of (his) life, a complete moron," and proceed to read what I find to be an articulate and insightful narrative, I realize how Kevin and I would measure his performance and intellect very differently. However, his yardstick ultimately frames his life experience. He gives some wonderful advice to others, to be kind and patient with themselves, but it is advice he himself has trouble heeding. It strikes me that during the course of our lives, we each have to modify our standards, and often, we reexamine some of our values. It usually is a gradual, lifelong process. We don't change so drastically on a daily basis as to no longer recognize ourselves, which I think is what has happened to Kevin. Maybe the suddenness with which Kevin has confronted change has made it especially difficult to adapt and to find himself.

"Addendum 2/18/96" Journal by Kevin

It is now late Saturday night with my absolutely boring and pathetic life, I decided to try and write a little of my thoughts. Mary Ann Bruce had ask me to think about publishing my story, which was written nearly three years ago. My first thought was if the story was to be published, it needs to be polished for a publishable condition. Further thoughts have contradicted this move. The story was written in the summer of 1993. It had many conditions and circumstances at that time. There have been many changes in 3 years. The conditions are much different now. To go back and change what is a "snap-shot" of time, would be falsifying the nativity of the scenario. It would not be just to present a different view. Realism must be the dominant factor for this writer. Therefore, I have decided to leave my original story alone, not look at it, and write an addendum to the story without the influence of seeing the original document. Here goes.

Like I stated above, 1995 was a year full of great mental and psychological challenges. To illustrate my point, it is necessary to be equipped with my general background information. Before my injury, I was one of those person that was very conscious of his goals, position in society, education, as well as money. In the least, I was very self-confident. A "Cocky" attitude is more like the correct adjective. After graduating with honors from high school, I went on to graduate with a bachelor degree in Electrical Engineering from (...name of university), which is well known nationally for their science program. During my professional career with an aerospace firm as a design engineer, I took on a new challenge to further my education. Thus, night-school for my M.B.A. while working full time during daylight hours. Soon after my graduation from MBA masters program, I started my own retail business. Equipped with only business training, I had to learn the ropes of business with the sharks on the streets. Four years later, I had my unfortunate head injury accident. Before the accident, as you can see, I was one of those people who gets things done once I put my mind to a certain task. It wasn't "if it can be done", it was "when will the goals be accomplished". Once I decided to do something, it would be done.

Two years after my incident, I decided to go back to (...name of university) to take a course, thus getting my feet wet again. At first, it was fun and well worth the effort. I did not encounter as much problems as I had anticipated. Somehow I had this delusion that I would continue college as the person I once was. I would get my P.H.D. in Business from (...name of university), name my college of choice to teach at, join the wonderful world of lecturing for a good living and retire. Some dream huh? My first obstacle was to take the entrance exam for the P.H.D program. As usual, I studied on my own and did not think I needed any preparation courses. Furthermore, I decided to take the entrance exam without any handicap perks. The testing administration gives handicapped individuals some extra perks, such as isolation rooms and additional testing time. I felt that if I was going to succeed, I must take the test as a member of the general population. Therefore, I would not dilute my final scores by taking advantage of what was offered to the disabled. I had very average results on the entrance exam, which would not be close to the scores needed for the selection committee at the university. Obviously disappointed, I struggled for weeks trying to cope mentally with the reality of the situation that I am now no longer the person I used to be. For the very first time, I had to realize the present situation. Even when I put my mind to a specific goal, the result was that someone or something told me I cannot accomplish that goal because I wasn't good enough. Wait one minute! This fact is something I never experience before. This was a tough aspect to handle because my ego as well as my self-esteem took a beating. It took me a long time to realize who I am now and move on. I still do not know what I should move-on to, but all I know is that if I keep my feet on the ground and always look around, I'm sure I will find something.

The second significant transformation in my thinking is that I am always uncomfortable at the thought of that something terribly wrong is going to occur. I do not possess the self confidence in myself that I used to. Therefore, I always think something bad is going to happen to me. This particular feeling is probably a result of a combination of factors, but I have not been able to pinpoint the exact contributing factor. No one should be living life on such constant pins and needles. Life is not meant to live as such. But that is the way I feel all the time. I sincerely hope I have expressed my feelings in a clear, understandable, concise and emphatic way.

Perhaps the ultimate psychological challenge is having to accept the fact that am now a very dependent person. I do not possess the self confidence to go out and take on life on my own. I need my close relatives to contribute to my own sense of survivability. I know for a fact that if something tragic were to happen to my wife, I would be the first person to fall apart at the scene. I don't know if I'm making any sense here, but going from an extremely independent person to someone that is very dependent on others is probably the toughest mental adjustment and challenge.

Where do I go from here? Not many people know exactly where the future would take them. Once, I had a clear vision of who and where I want to be. Not anymore. Am I afraid and sadden by this fact? Of course I am! At times, I'm bitter too. However, I will always remember that the uncertainty of life is what makes it fun and worth living.

Discussion Questions

1. Discuss and give examples of the constraints on letting patients/clients "do it their way."
2. How would you respond to Kevin's description of his testing and application to graduate school?
3. Discuss Kevin's feelings about being dependent. How are these similar or different from your feelings about being dependent?
4. Compare "Addendum 2/18/96" to his original (1993) story and identify what, if any, changes you perceive in Kevin's values, perceptions of himself, feelings, and goals.

Impressions

MAB: Kevin's most recent entry calls my attention to changes in Kevin's writing, feelings, and beliefs as well as some stable features. He continues to have high expectations for himself, wishes no special considerations, and values living and the fun of challenge. He evaluates his status relative to dependence-independence and talks about the emotional impact of his feeling dependent. Sometimes, in rehabilitation, I feel that we focus so much on helping people regain independence that we fail to help patients realistically adjust to the dependence necessitated by their disability. Nor do we consider that there are positions of dependence, interdependence, and independence in all of our lives.

Like many patients I have treated, Kevin wishes no special considerations. I respect his as well as others' standards, but these standards can defeat a person. This seems to be the case in Kevin's testing situation. I guess this is one of the major challenges in therapy: how to help a patient meet his or her standards or adjust them when his or her performance ability is limited or absent. I have had patients get angry, give up, feel helpless, or find fault with therapy. Kevin, although disappointed, is looking to "move-on" and is "sure (he) will find something." As a therapist, I want to support his optimism, but I am at a loss for options that I feel would be acceptable to Kevin. I don't think he would, at this time, consider options of test preparation, retesting under special conditions, or applying to a different institution. I can help him move on and explore other goals, but Kevin's values influence his choices and we need to work within his value system. The challenge in therapy is to help patients learn from their failures or disappointments and match their values and abilities to set and achieve goals. With Kevin, I might try using his rules for living in which he refers to learning in "...the full-time informal school called life." I can encourage him to use what he has learned as he "moves-on." However, my gut feeling is that Kevin needs to explore on his own and do it his way, a need many patients have.

BB: Fine (1993) writes that "...the most stressful dimensions of trauma and illness are often those that challenge personal assumptions about one's self..." (p. 17). Three years later in Kevin's journal he closes with, "Once, I had a clear vision of who and where I want to be. Not anymore." The challenge is still around personal visions. He continues to measure himself by uncompromising yardsticks. In the "Addendum 2/18/96," we see this when he writes about being "dependent" (viewed negatively) rather than "independent" (viewed positively). There seems to be no in-between.

I was especially taken with Kevin's recognition that he is "always uncomfortable at the thought that something terribly wrong is going to occur." If I put his "Addendum 2/18/96" with Kevin's original material, his story starts to take a slightly different shape for me. It becomes the story of someone who felt himself to be invincible who now feels very vulnerable. I wonder to what extent feeling vulnerable is what many of our clients, and their families, seek protection from—and it's protection we can't give them. Recalling some of our earlier stories, perhaps it underlies the need clients have to control, or their wish that professionals behave as experts or give guarantees. Vulnerability—it's such a basic human condition.

"A Spouse's Point of View (1996)" by Polly

When I first read my husband's journal (story), I was saddened by his words of depression, frustration, disappointment, and lack of confidence. During his recovery, he experienced many periods of deep depression and frustration. I felt hopeless in helping him cope with these depressive thoughts, mainly because there was, and still is, no way that I could ever possibly know what he was/is going through in trying to cope with his disabilities. I, too, constantly compared his recovery progress to how he was before the accident, which, as Kevin said, is the number one mistake that leads to disappointment.

I quickly began to realize, however, that his writing was a form of therapy for dealing with his depression. I began to see the positives instead of focusing on the negatives. With all that he had been through, the mere fact that he could sit down at a computer and express his thoughts and feelings in understandable words was in my mind a miracle. Looking back at it all, the writing of his journal (story) definitely served a unique purpose in his psychological rehabilitation process. It was his way of recognizing and accepting his disabilities, and identifying ways of living or adjusting to his new life. At the same time, his journal (story) provided me with new insight on the numerous psychological issues that he was trying to cope with. In my mind, Kevin's journal (story) provides a unique example of how a person's psychological rehabilitation progresses into acceptance and identification of adjustment for a new life.

Discussion Questions

1. What role might occupational therapy take in educating and supporting families of people with long-term disabilities?
2. Describe occupational therapy's participation in programs you have observed in which family education and support was a primary goal.
3. Discuss methods or strategies for getting feedback about a patient's/client's performance at home without violating patient-spouse confidentiality and trust.
4. Discuss and identify possible uses for journals in occupational therapy. Describe specific adaptations for chosen populations.
5. How might an occupational therapist respond to issues of dependence-interdependence-independence in therapy? Give examples, if you can, of specific tasks and therapist approaches.

Impressions

MAB: The feelings of helplessness Polly describes are similar to those expressed by family members and caregivers. This sense of helplessness and responsibility for the spouse's or family member's well-being frequently leads significant others to seek suggestions from staff. Clinicians give suggestions and may expect a great deal from significant others, whether for direct participation in treatment, follow through with protocols at home, or feedback about the patient's performance at home. While these expectations usually are met, even welcomed, they can add another burden to an overload of responsibility. Sometimes they also cause friction between the patient or client and the family member. For example, I have had patients who do not want their spouse to assume a therapist role, while others welcome the extra therapy time or assistance. Some patients resent that family members are giving staff feedback about their conduct. I can't count the times I've heard a patient exclaim, "Did he/she tell on me?" or "Don't you tell on me!"

Polly describes the disappointment that comes from comparing Kevin now to "how he was before the accident." I don't think that this can be avoided because patients as well as family members make comparisons. In fact, patients describe to me how they used to be, and may bring in pictures of themselves prior to their accident. Comparisons of function and lifestyle can help the therapist during evaluation and treatment. However, focusing on current performance and possibilities helps the patient transition to establishing a "new life."

Unlike some family members, Polly is able to focus on Kevin's "strengths" and tries to see the "positives." In my experience, this is a challenge for family members, especially if the patient emphasizes his or her limitations, losses, and inabilities. In that case, patients and clients may interpret support or one's identifying his or her strengths as a lack of sensitivity around his or her loss and disability. In many situations, a spouse or parent is key to helping a client see his or her strengths, because spouses and parents are so intimately involved in helping the client initiate tasks at home or return to activities outside of the home.

Polly shares her perception that keeping a journal has been very therapeutic for Kevin. In many settings, patients are encouraged to keep a journal as a form of cognitive rehabilitation, memory assist, or vehicle for self-expression and reflection (similar to the traditional diaries people keep). The journals take many forms. Patients may create their own structure. Kevin uses a narrative format and the computer. Others may use a looseleaf binder or a decorative book. Unlike Kevin, some people are unable to or have difficulty keeping a journal. Difficulties arise from limited written communication skills, poor visual motor skills, decreased attention, and reasons unique to patient interests and specific disabilities. When therapists use journals for specific therapeutic reasons, they need to be sensitive to patient needs and adapt the task accordingly. Patients frequently ask me what to include in their journal. An example of an adaptation of a journal is the "memory book" described by Dougherty and Radomski (1987). Their approach is influenced by memory research and their clinical experiences. They provide sample structures for a memory book and describe the role of the therapist in structuring the book, motivating patients to use it, and structuring practice for memory training. I also have seen adaptations of this format to allow patients to use computers, pictures to minimize narrative entries, or entries from therapists and significant others.

BB: Polly's initial feelings of sadness and hopelessness, and her concern that she might only partially understand all that Kevin has gone through, echoes similar feelings voiced by many family members I have known. I believe there is special agony experienced by individuals who witness a person they love in pain. Many will say, "It would be better if it were me (going through this illness or disability)." Parents hurt for their children, spouses for each other, children for their parents. Sometimes this generates feelings of guilt: "I shouldn't have a good day if (this person I love) is having a bad day" or "I shouldn't feel sorry for myself, because look at all he/she has to go through." There is usually much sadness, frustration, and anger before some kind of equanimity can be achieved. For each client we encounter there are many like Polly, whom we may or may not meet, whose lives are irrevocably changed.

In "Kevin's Rules for Living," he writes, "There is no part of life that does not contain lessons." We again wish to thank Kevin and Polly and our other contributors for what they have shared and for allowing us to learn from their stories.

References

Dougherty, P.M., & Radomski, M.V. (1987). *The cognitive rehabilitation workbook: A systematic approach to improving independent living skills in brain-injured adults.* Rockville, MD: Aspen Publications.

Fine, S. (1993). Interaction between psychological variables and cognitive function. In C.B. Royeen (Ed.), *AOTA self-study series: Cognitive rehabilitation.* Rockville, MD: American Occupational Therapy Association.

Glaser, B., & Strauss, A. (1967). *The discovery of grounded theory: Strategies for qualitative research.* Chicago: Aldine.

Strauss, A., & Corbin, J. (1994). Grounded theory methodology: An overview. In N.K. Denzin & Y.S. Lincoln (Eds.), *Handbook of qualitative research.* Thousand Oaks, CA: Sage Publications.

Index

For your information

This book and many others on numerous different topics are available from SLACK Incorporated. For further information or a copy of our latest catalog, contact us at:

Professional Book Division
SLACK Incorporated
6900 Grove Road
Thorofare, NJ 08086 USA
Telephone: 1-609-848-1000
1-800-257-8290
Fax: 1-609-853-5991
E-mail: orders@slackinc.com
WWW: http://www.slackinc.com

We accept most major credit cards and checks or money orders in US dollars drawn on a US bank. Most orders are shipped within 72 hours.

Contact us for information on recent releases, forthcoming titles, and bestsellers. If you have a comment about this title or see a need for a new book, direct your correspondence to the Editorial Director at the above address.

If you are an instructor, we can be reached at the address listed above or on the Internet at ***educomps@slackinc.com*** *for specific needs.*

Thank you for your interest and we hope you found this work beneficial.